BREAKING *the* SILENCE

Recovering from Miscarriage, Stillbirth, & Early Neonatal Death

Sylvia E. Sheets McDonald

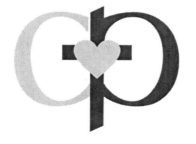

CarePoint Ministries ❖ *Atlanta*
www.ChristianCarePoint.org

CarePoint Ministries, Inc.
A faith-based publishing ministry
www.CarePointMinistry.org
Atlanta, GA USA

CarePoint titles are available at discounts in bulk quantities. For details, contact the publisher at the above address.

Printed and Manufactured in the United States of America

Important Note: If at any time you feel you need to speak with a pastoral or professional Christian counselor, please call the church office for a referral to a member of our pastoral staff or a licensed professional Christian counselor. Church telephone number:

_____

Dedication

This workbook is dedicated to all my children...

To my two beautiful daughters, Sara and Katie who were taken from me all too soon. While you were unknown to the world, you were so well known by me and fully known by our Creator. Thank you for teaching me how precious life is and about being a mother.

For my son, Evan, thank you for being everything I always dreamed my son would be; and Seth, thank you for being everything I never knew I dreamed of in a son. To my little girl, Abigail, may you always be as true to yourself as you are now...I'm so proud of who you are.

And finally, thank you Lord, for allowing me to know and love these precious people and giving me the privilege of calling them "my child."

Acknowledgements

First, I want to thank my dear husband, John, who always tried to do what he felt was best for me at all times. I thank God every day for such a wonderful, Christian man. And, for giving me the blessing of having you as a husband.

To my Mom, who's the strongest person I know. Thank you for showing me, by example, what a "Mom" is supposed to be. I know your love for me is second only to His.

To my Dad for always giving me everything he could. You're a wonderful father and grandfather and we are all so blessed to have you in our lives.

Christa, thank you for sharing your talent with me, and more importantly, your friendship.

Dave, the best pastor in the world, thank you for giving me sound, Biblical teaching…not to mention friendship.

My "first editor," Destiny, what would I have ever done without your input, encouragement, and flawless punctuation skills? You're the best.

Evan, Seth and Abby…thank you for always being a wonderful inspiration…in more ways than you could possibly imagine.

Finally, thank you Jesus for not only carrying me when I couldn't walk, but for holding me up when I couldn't even stand.

Contents

Introduction

Did you know that one in four pregnancies ends in miscarriage or stillbirth? (Goldback). And these are the ones after the positive pregnancy test! Some researchers estimate that as many as 40% of all conceptions end in miscarriage, many before a woman takes a pregnancy test (Lasker and Toedter, 2000). While these are alarming statistics, it is much more alarming when one realizes that with these statistics, the support given to those suffering from pregnancy loss is vitally lacking.

Some will state another vital statistic to remedy the incompatibility that exists between lack of support verses the high occurrence of loss. They will state that 80% of miscarriages are termed "single miscarriages." This means that the vast majority of women can expect a normal, healthy pregnancy the second time they conceive. However, the fact that the woman grieves her first child is lost in the statistic. Also, the fact that neonatal loss "happens to many, many women" is also irrelevant. You lost YOUR baby. That's really all that matters.

Grief following miscarriage is usually intense and traumatic. It's a sudden shock to the system: physically, spiritually and emotionally. A once joyful day, filled with bright and hopeful anticipation and excitement, is suddenly ripped apart by words like "there's no longer a heartbeat," when you see blood, or feel those horrible cramping pains. Immediately, a woman kicks into "mama bear mode" and knows, deep in her gut, that something is horribly wrong. And still, some people don't call her a mother. It's clear that she's a mother, just by her instincts.

Ironically, this sudden tragedy often gets overlooked by society. Grieving couples are told to "move on," forget or are simply ignored altogether. Grief is hard enough to handle

Grief following miscarriage is usually intense and traumatic. It's a sudden shock to the system: physically, spiritually and emotionally.

It's time to break the silence of grief and share with those who have "walked a mile in your shoes."

alone. Lack of understanding and information haunt today's population. Social isolation and silence only make it worse.

Before the "Internet Age," grieving parents were left alone. And alone they stayed, without help or support. Now, with the world of internet interaction, many online web sites offer support communities (see page 107 for more information). This has made the world of grief from miscarriage, stillbirth, and early neonatal loss a little bit smaller, a little tighter. However, there is still something about real, live people looking into your face, seeing your tears and saying "you're not alone." That's exactly why we're here. That's exactly why this was created. It's time to break the silence of grief and share with those who have "walked a mile in your shoes." The others in this group have felt the same burning pain of loss, the same social isolation and seek the same validation that you do. You are not alone.

Miscarriage, Stillbirth, Early Neonatal Grief

America's attitude and awareness on grief and death received enlightenment when Elizabeth Kubler-Ross released her work on grief and bereavement in 1969. Her main contribution was her description on the stages of grief. For those suffering "specialized grief" such as those of us dealing with the loss of a child in-utero or shortly thereafter, it's paralleled to that of the loss of any dear loved one and to any other parent who loses a child, despite the age of that child.

What are the symptoms of parental grief?

1. Sadness

2. Yearning for the lost child

3. Desire to talk with others about their loss/their child

4. Desire for meaningful explanation/information about their loss

What are the marked differences with miscarriage/stillbirth/early neonatal grief?

1. Lack of rituals (no burial or memorial services)

2. Lack of community understanding/sympathy

3. Perceived guilt due to "failure to carry the baby" to term

Spiritual Aspects

The tragic, premature death of a baby can wreak havoc on the spiritual health of a parent. One might often blame God for the death. "You could have stopped this!" a parent might cry out to the heavens. Anger and resentment can easily build up between you and your Savior.

It's also natural for a grieving parent to simply want God to answer the question "Why?" Without an immediate, clear-cut answer, the parent again begins to build up walls to block out Biblical truths and principles in his/her life. While striving to fulfill the desire to know why, God is often pushed aside.

Sadly, one of the most hurtful responses, "Your baby is in heaven with God; he's in a better place now," can often lead a grieving parent to resentment. While we want to shout out, from the depths of our very being, "I want my child here, with me!" we usually put on a mask and say "I know," and continue on with life. By allowing this type of frustration to build, we allow the enemy to consume our grief and push us farther away from the One who wants to comfort us the most.

Social Aspects

Grieving from the loss of a child almost always ensures a time of isolation. This can occur in our homes, churches and workplace. Often lack of understanding and knowledge lead people to say the wrong thing to a grieving parent or to say nothing at all. Parents who grieve "unborn children" are often called "silent grievers"—their grief is not socially acceptable.

Society as a whole takes the "get over it and get on with it" attitude to those suffering from grief after a miscarriage, stillbirth or early neonatal death. Grief is not allowed past a socially acceptable time frame set up by those around us. Excuses are made by others as to why we should not be still grieving. The lost child is never discussed and the parent is left alone.

Often the griever's family is of no comfort. They, too, lack understanding as to what to say and do. Unless they've experienced a similar loss, it's hard for them to comprehend your grief. The dead child is no longer a child to them and is simply a memory of what once was but never materialized. To the parents, they've lost a child...to the family, they only lost a dream.

Sadly, many marriages don't make it through such difficult times. Studies show that the mother's grief is oftentimes

Sadly, one of the most hurtful responses, "Your baby is in heaven with God; he's in a better place now" can often lead a grieving parent to resentment.

Society as a whole takes the "get over it and get on with it" attitude to those suffering from grief after a miscarriage, stillbirth or early neonatal death.

more complex and lasts longer than the father's. Since everyone's grief is unique, it needs to be viewed as such. However, lack of understanding often drives a wedge between the married couple. Lack of communication begins to erode the foundation of their marriage until it finally breaks, leaving shambles. Therefore, it is essential that couples who find they are struggling during this time seek professional counseling to work through their grief individually as well as a couple.

Psychological/Mental Aspects

The psychological aspects after the loss of a child are vast and devastating. A mother and father are usually riddled with fear, grief, guilt, anger and despair. The range of emotions is almost endless.

> Psychologically, an attachment has occurred between the parents and the baby. This attachment has taken place despite the fact that the parent has never actually seen the baby.

Psychologically, an attachment has occurred between the parents and the baby. This attachment has taken place despite the fact that the parent has never actually seen the baby. Simply knowing that the baby is there, via a positive pregnancy test, is enough to begin to create the bond. With each passing day the bond becomes stronger and more established. We form a mental image of our child...what he or she will look like, what name we will give the baby, and we also talk to our baby. Suddenly taking that away is a tragic, horrific death.

Bereavement is usually defined by three responses. First is shock and numbness. This usually occurs after the news has been delivered that the baby has died. The second is a yearning and pining for the deceased. Parents want their babies. This is natural. This is usually accompanied with a preoccupation of the baby as well. The last is depression and disorganization. The parent's world is turned upside-down and he/she is left to pick up the pieces.

There are also multi-dimensional components to grief. Lasker and Toedter (2000), used three stages to address the specific grief suffered by those experiencing loss due to a miscarriage or stillbirth. The first is Active Grief. This involves sadness, crying for the baby, and missing the baby. The second is labeled Difficulty Coping. This involves difficulty in dealing with normal activities and with people. It also indicates withdrawal and depression. The third is despair. This stage is characterized by worthlessness and hopelessness.

Research has proposed that the grief and shock following the loss of a child qualifies for classification under post-traumatic stress disorder or more specifically, "traumatic grief" as proposed by Prigerson (1999). The key element that separates traumatic grief from post traumatic stress is in the case of traumatic grief, there is a preoccupation with the deceased child and a feeling of being "stunned." This distinction between traumatic grief and post traumatic stress is significant as it allows management of depressive symptoms as well as focused therapy when needed. At times, depending on the individual reaction to the loss and his/her coping skills, intense counseling might be the best means used as opposed to support groups. Should you feel as if you need such focused counseling, especially if you feel suicidal, please seek professional help as outlined in this workbook (see pages 3 and 107).

Self Rating Scale

Below is a modified checklist for you to do a self rating to see if you may be suffering from grief, and more specifically, what stage of grief you are in presently. This is a very simple and quick check and by no means exhaustive. Simply circle the number that corresponds: 5 Strongly Agree, 4 Agree, 3 Neutral, 2 Disagree, 1 Strongly Disagree.

This is a very simple and quick check and by no means exhaustive.

1. I feel sad	5	4	3	2	1
2. Most people annoy me	5	4	3	2	1
3. I feel empty	5	4	3	2	1
4. I can't perform daily tasks	5	4	3	2	1
5. I want to talk about my baby	5	4	3	2	1
6. I'm fearful	5	4	3	2	1
7. I've thought about suicide	5	4	3	2	1
8. I feel I need counseling for my grief	5	4	3	2	1
9. I don't feel like I'm moving on	5	4	3	2	1
10. I cry a lot	5	4	3	2	1
11. I feel guilty	5	4	3	2	1
12. I don't want to go out	5	4	3	2	1
13. I feel worthless since he/she died	5	4	3	2	1
14. I'm not living, just "existing"	5	4	3	2	1
15. I worry about the future	5	4	3	2	1
16. I'm lonely	5	4	3	2	1

17. My friends and family let me down	5	4	3	2	1
18. Thinking about my loss is very painful	5	4	3	2	1

Scoring

Add up the numbers in the following groups:

Active Grief: Numbers 1, 3, 5, 6, 10, 18

Difficulty Coping: Numbers 2, 4, 8, 12, 16, 17

Despair: Numbers 7, 9, 11, 13, 14, 15

The group with the highest number should show you the stage of grief you are currently experiencing.

So where's God in all of this?

God is right in the middle of all of this, whether you know it or not. God sheds your tears. His Holy Spirit intercedes for you with groans when you don't have the right words to pray. When you're feeling your loneliest, he's right there, carrying you.

Spiritual Warfare

Satan loves it when we hurt. Rest assured that he's delighting in this now. He watches and waits, longing for the right opportunity to exploit you and the memory of your baby.

Satan once had a foothold on this area. Death separated us from God. Jesus died so that while we were all still sinners, we would have life again, through him. Jesus made it possible for us to be reunited once again with our beloved child. Don't let Satan take that way from you or distort it in any way.

Satan will also work through others, even the ones you love the most. Vulnerability is a tool that he loves to use. If you have gaping wounds exposed, he will smell the blood. Does this mean you should hide the grief or suppress it? By no means! What this means is that if your wounds are freshly opened by those whom you love the most, there will be a two-pronged effect. First, the wound itself is vulnerable. For example, when you hear the words "You should be over this grieving by now; it's already been a month," you have the wound opened and exposed that says "I'm grieving, and it's not validated by others"; and second, you have the perception of "I'm so alone. Why aren't they more understanding?" This makes you vulnerable to even more devastating sadness and anger. Satan loves this type of vulnerability and will use

Satan loves it when we hurt. Rest assured that he's delighting in this now.

this to drive a wedge between you, your family, your friends and your Savior.

Depression is another tool that Satan loves to use. Depression leaves us weak and tired. It makes us feel worthless and without hope. Hell is depression. It's a total separation from God where there is no hope, no light. During your depression, Satan will fill your mind with various ill-conceived thoughts. "If God loved you, your baby wouldn't have died. You must have made him mad. You deserve this." Another might be "go ahead and end your life, then you can be with your baby again." Don't let Satan convince you. Use your Bible and your prayers to communicate the truth. Allowing yourself to entertain these ideas will only lead you to more lies and give more control to the enemy.

What does the Bible say?

Grief is spoken of many times in the Bible. God grieved. Those whom he dearly loves grieve. Jesus grieved. It is acceptable. For everything, there is a time. Your time to grieve is right now.

First, it's critical to see that our Creator grieved. Genesis 6:6 says "The Lord was grieved…in his heart." God was grieving because his creation had separated themselves from him. He mourned the loss of the close relationship he had with Adam and Eve in the garden, and then he mourned over the wickedness of his creation in the times of Noah. He grieved because his children had been separated from him. Evil consumed the hearts of man instead of love for the one who had given life, and they sought him not. His heart broke, just as yours is breaking. The Creator knows your pain and grief.

The Creator knows your pain and grief.

Jesus too, spoke of his grief. First, he wept at the death of Lazarus. He felt the sting caused by death. He knew that he would one day conquer death but still felt the sadness of loss. He would revisit that place later in life while praying in the garden before his crucifixion.

Luke 22:42 shows Jesus pleading, "Father if you are willing, please take this cup from me." He didn't want to die. Even though the Savior knew how it would all end, he still asked the Father to let him avoid death. Death is always painful, even if not for the deceased. The wounds it leaves behind in the flesh of those we love always create memorial scars. Jesus further went on praying, and in verse 44 we read that "being in anguish…sweat like drops of blood were falling to the ground." Medical explanation suggests that these were actual drops of blood that occur when under extreme stress—a person's capillaries burst, causing one to "sweat blood." Jesus knew death. And he knew grief.

Furthermore, Jesus knew loneliness and lack of understanding. While praying in the garden, Jesus took his three closest and dearest friends. He simply asked them to stay awake, keep watch and pray. None of them did. He was left alone. He would return over and over again, only to find them sleeping. They didn't understand, and he was alone. He even pleaded with them saying "my heart is overwhelmed with sorrow, to the point of death." We understand what he means, we've felt it too. But his friends didn't. So they slept, leaving him to grieve alone.

Finally, I think we need to look at the hope that the Bible offers. It is not known why things happen the way they do, and it's not for us to decide and interpret. Human nature presses us on to answer the question "why?" Sadly, the simple matter of fact is that we live in a fallen world. Sin consumes it. Tragic things happen to everyone, even those that love and serve the Lord. Consequently, his word gives us promise.

Hope abounds throughout his words. Paul faces horrible challenges and still gives God his praise. He says "when I am weak, then I am strong" (2 Corinthians 12:10), knowing that he must rely on God when life is toughest. Job's story also stands out. He lost everything: wealth, love and friendship. He lost those he loved the most. And, he persevered through his grief, learning from it and being stronger on the other side.

Hope is offered throughout the Bible. The book of Psalms is an excellent source of hope. I strongly advise you to read through this book as you go through your grief. Allow it to invade your very being, just as your grief has. 2 Corinthians 4:8-9, 16 says, "we are hard pressed on every side, but not crushed; perplexed, but not in despair, persecuted but not abandoned; struck down, but not destroyed...Therefore, we do not lose heart. Though outwardly we are wasting away, yet inwardly, we are being renewed day by day." *What a blessed hope!*

We can take reassurance in the fact that God has a plan for our lives, one that will never harm us (Jeremiah 29). We need to surrender it to him. Is that an easy task while we grieve? Usually not. Grieving is a process that needs to be walked through. You will literally "walk through the valley of the

We can take reassurance in the fact that God has a plan for our lives, one that will never harm us (Jeremiah 29).

shadow of death," but do not fear. He is with you. Allow him to comfort you by reading his word daily, praying for surrender and forgiveness, and for healing. Remember, the only way to deal with grief is to go through it. Suppressing it, ignoring it or denying it will only allow it to fester like an infected thorn in your side. Acknowledge it, confront it and deal with it.

Practical Suggestions in Dealing with Grief

The only way to deal with grief is to go through it. Here are some helpful suggestions that should allow you to begin healing after suffering the trauma of losing your child.

❶ Acknowledge your grief. If you wear the "Yes, I'm doing fine" mask all day, you will eventually be exhausted beyond belief. It is essentially like trying to live a lie. It doesn't do yourself or your child's memory any justice. Eventually, the grief will surface. By acknowledging your grief right away, you begin the healing process.

❷ Discuss your grief. Being in a support group such as this is a wonderful step. Individual and couples counseling is also very beneficial. Communication is key in understanding and support.

❸ Let go of the guilt. A crucial step in dealing with the grief of losing a child through miscarriage and stillbirth is realizing that your child's death was not your fault. We all want to point a finger at someone, usually we point at ourselves for blame. Let go of this guilt.

❹ Experience the anger, let it go, offer forgiveness. Anger is a natural and normal response to the loss of a baby. Experience this, but don't dwell on it. Satan loves to work through anger. Remember that while we were still sinners, Christ forgave us. It is our duty to do the same.

❺ Healing takes time. Grieving parents are often asked years after their babies die "does it get easier?" Most will answer "No, it just gets more manageable." You will never forget the child you lost, nor should you. But be patient with yourself and your grief. God will work with you through this. Go to him daily and ask for his arms to cradle you.

❻ Rely on your support systems. Asking for additional help is always a sign of strength. If you feel that you

The only way to deal with grief is to go through it.

need more in-depth counseling, seek it. If you feel like you simply need a shoulder to cry on for that day, seek it. There are many health care professionals, pastors, lay members, friends and family who would be more than happy to help you. You just need to ask.

For a list of supportive resources and organizations, see *Where to Go for Help* at the back of this workbook.

A Plan of His Own

"'For I know the plans I have for you,' declares the Lord, 'plans to prosper you and not to harm you, plans to give you hope and a future.'"

—Jeremiah 29:11

"'You will seek me and find me when you seek me with all your heart.'"

—Jeremiah 29:13

Welcome & Purpose

Welcome to Breaking the Silence support group. This group is for people dealing with grief due to miscarriage and stillbirth. The purpose of the group is to:

share the love, grace and mercy of Christ Jesus. We'll accomplish this by sharing and bearing one another's burdens, expressing our love and care for one another, and encouraging one another so that we might find peace, calm and joy.

Opening Prayer

Dear God,

Thank you for giving us all the courage and strength to join this group. We honestly seek your presence, guidance, love and comfort. We ask that you guide our meeting tonight as we get to know one another through our shared stories, fears, hopes and grief. Allow us to bear witness to each other's life in a way that allows us to carry each other's burdens. Help us to allow others to carry ours. Thank you for carrying our burdens. Thank you for who you are and what you will do through this group.

In Jesus' name,
Amen.

❶ Since the heart of a small group is interaction, take a moment to introduce yourself to everyone. If you feel comfortable, briefly state what brought you to this meeting (meaning, briefly describe your recent/past loss). (In the space below you may want to jot a note or two as each member shares. This will also allow you to understand the stage of grief each person/couple might be facing.)

_____

_____

_____

_____

_____

Our Group Covenant

This group is a covenant group. Covenants help us to build trust, share openly, and love and care for each other on the hills and in the valleys of our lives.

Agreeing to a covenant for our group at the outset is important. Your group shepherd will provide you with a sample covenant. As a group you can do with it as you will: adopt it as it is, adopt it and adapt it, or scrap it and draft your own from scratch.

A Plan of His Own

Someone volunteer to read or play the companion cd.

"'For I know the plans I have for you,' declares the Lord, 'plans to prosper you and not to harm you, plans to give you hope and a future.'"

—*Jeremiah 29:11*

"'You will seek me and find me when you seek me with all your heart.'"

—*Jeremiah 29:13*

"Okay, you have to push now," she said.

"No, I can't. It's too early. You know they can't survive if they're born now. It's too early. It's too early," I said.

Gently, the nurse took my hand. I could see the worn gold cross that hung on a chain from around her neck as if it was there to remind me of the prayer that I had lifted to God just hours before.

"Honey," she said softly, "they're already gone. You need to deliver these babies' bodies now. Their spirits are gone. They are already with God in heaven."

The sobering thought ran up my spine. The machine beside me signaled that the contractions were constant and hard, but I was too numb to feel the pain. I looked away from her necklace, then to the machine, then to the Bible that sat on the nightstand beside the hospital bed. While nurses ran about the room, monitors beeped and surgical instruments were being prepared for delivery. Amidst all the chaos, I lay there gazing at my Bible.

This was the same Bible that I had since I gave my life to God during opening convention at college my freshman year. I went with my college roommate the day after and bought it at the bookstore. It was the first Bible I bought and the first one I ever read—the first one I ever wanted to read. It had highlighted verses, dog-eared pages and notes scribbled in the margins. It looked like it was about 50 years old and had been through a battle zone. In reality, it was only four years old.

I drank the words in that worn book. It sat on my night stand while I slept, and I carried it in my backpack when I was awake. In it I read about Moses, Noah, Jeremiah, John, Peter, Paul and Jesus. I learned of God's promises, his mercy, his plans, and his will. Most importantly, I learned of his love for me, his love for us all.

I had read verses in it that said "Surely the righteous…are rewarded" (Psalm 58:11). This is where I had started two days before, but not at all where I had ended.

Two days earlier, while getting ready to go meet my parents for dinner, my water broke. I literally flooded the floors in our house from the amniotic fluid I had accumulated in just five short months. I had experienced a very bad pregnancy filled with constant illness, swelling and pain. Yet, I was told that it was all "normal" for a twin pregnancy and that I should just deal with the "inconveniences" until my delivery. Suddenly, my delivery was here, way too early, at only 21 weeks and 5 days gestation.

Upon arrival at the hospital, I was told by the doctor that my labor could probably be stopped. However, since my water broke, there was little else they could do medically for my babies unless miraculously, the tear in the amniotic sac

"Honey," she said softly, "they're already gone. You need to deliver these babies' bodies now...."

healed. The nurse who admitted me into the hospital told me bluntly, "All you can really do now is pray." And pray is exactly what I did.

Immediately, my husband and I asked the Lord to save our babies. We asked him to heal the tear and allow it to fill with amniotic fluid. We asked for protection against germs and other diseases that the twins could contract now that their protection from the outside world was broken. We prayed for God's peace. We read scripture from my Bible that comforted us.

Once the word spread that I was in the hospital, I was blessed with many visitors. Most all of them prayed with me and asked for God to help me carry these babies to term. Many prayed, asking for God's help in delivering two healthy babies into this world. Several ministers whom I knew from college and local churches prayed with me, again, asking God to be with me and for him to protect my babies and help them to be born healthy and strong. My Christian friends and family offered up the same prayer on my behalf. Everyone prayed for this tear to be healed.

After everyone left on the second night, I lifted my old, familiar Bible from the night stand. I prayed for the Lord to guide me through the study of his Word and for him to comfort me through scripture. I opened the Bible to the Lord's prayer and began to read. Suddenly, I realized that I had left a crucial element out of my prayers, and so had everyone else. I had not asked for "God's will to be done." How could we have all forgotten this? I wondered.

Almost chilling to me was the abrupt realization that God's will might be for the tear not to heal or even for my children not to survive. Immediately, I put the thought out of my mind. God loves me and loves my children, so why would he want them to die? That's ridiculous, I thought. Yet, I could not bring myself to pray "Your will be done, Father." Besides, I was not ready to close with prayer yet, so I kept reading.

Again, putting the thought out of my mind, I rationalized that this scripture reading was just a "fluke" and that I just happened to come across it and it must mean something else for me. So I decided to read something from the Old Testament instead.

Turning randomly to Jeremiah, I began reading on what seemed to be safe territory. After reading the first two pages that I had chosen, I turned the page to one that had been

> Almost chilling to me was the abrupt realization that God's will might be for the tear not to heal or even for my children not to survive.

dog-eared several times and had a verse highlighted in bright pink and underlined repeatedly. In the side margin read these words scribbled in my own handwriting:

"Sylvia, never forget this promise that God has made to you!" and it pointed back to very familiar verses in Jeremiah 29:11 and 13, "'For I know the plans I have for you,' declares the Lord, 'plans to prosper you and not to harm you, plans to give you hope and a future...You will seek me and find me when you seek me with all your heart.'"

God had led me here in scripture and I had found him. Closing my eyes, with tears streaming down my face, I realized what I had to do. I prayed "Father, may your will be done in my life and in the lives of these two babies. You know the plans for our lives, and I know that they are what is best for us. I give my life to you, and my children are yours. Amen."

Those words and the memory of that moment echoed in my mind as I stared at that worn Bible sitting beside my hospital bed. My trance was snapped by the cross necklace that I had just seen a moment before. The nurse was standing between me and the night stand. Gently, she put her hand on my arm and said "Your husband is on his way but you are beginning to deliver one of the twins now. Her head is crowning so you need to push to fully deliver her. The time has come."

She was right. The time had come for God's will to be done in our lives. The prayer that I had prayed two hours earlier was heard and God's plan for my life was at hand. I had finally sought him with all of my heart. I came to realize that I had a plan, but God, my Father, had a plan of his own. My children were stillborn shortly thereafter.

I did not know the reason why God's plan meant that my children would not survive. I didn't know why I carried them to 22 weeks or why I endured 22 weeks of illness carrying them. I didn't know why I was blessed with their presence in my life, albeit brief. I didn't know why some are healed and why some, like me, were not.

What I do know is that God's plan for me is just that, his plan. I know that when I seek him with all of my heart, I am in his will, and above all, that is where I want to be. I know that his will and his plans for me and my life will never harm me and that I have a hope and a future in him. Most importantly, I know that he loves me. And at that moment, that's all I really needed to know.

> I did not know the reason why God's plan meant that my children would not survive. I didn't know why I carried them to 22 weeks....

What I didn't know was that all I thought I knew was about to be tested, and all the emotions I had ever felt in my life were about to be revisited, only this time, in a vibrant, passionate, and disturbing way. While I thought God had unfolded his plan for me at that moment, it was only the beginning of a very long journey...one that I still walk today.

Passage Comments

This is the first introduction to my story. Yours might be similar in some aspects and completely different in others. The commonality that binds you with me is that you and I are grieving the death of a child. It has been said that "there are no coffins for the unborn." I know and understand the pain that comes with that statement alone—a statement that only those who have traveled this journey understand.

It may appear as if I'm confident and secure in my faith and my love of my Savior. Ironically, throughout the next sessions you will see that I will come full circle away from it and then back again. This is my grief story. Yours might mirror it, or be completely different. The main focus here will be allowing yourself to share your grief among those who understand it.

Discussion

❶ Look back over the story. Have you asked yourself and/or God similar questions? Explain.

_____

_____

_____

_____

_____

❷ What do you think the author will experience next?

_____

_____

_____

_____

❸ What did you experience after you realized you would not be taking your child home from the hospital?

_____

_____

_____

_____

❹ When you realized you were losing your child, did you feel close to God or far away from him?

_____

_____

_____

_____

❺ Do you think the author's optimistic outlook on what was happening to her will continue? Why or why not?

_____

_____

_____

_____

❻ What do you think her husband was experiencing during this time? Do you think his perspective was different? Explain.

_____

_____

_____

_____

_____

In this group, the words "I understand" take on a whole new meaning. Too often these words come frequently from those who try to comfort, but really cannot understand the pain and grief of losing a child. The others in this group may be the closest thing to "understanding" that you will ever know. Allow this understanding to flourish in your heart.

Reflection

Take some time on your own, outside of the group time, to journal about your thoughts on this chapter.

_____

_____

_____

_____

_____

_____

_____

_____

_____

_____

_____

_____

Encouragement

"Jesus invites us to come, as we are when we are tired of life and burdened down by the things that make no sense. He calls us to come when we are angry and confused. Jesus calls us to come to Him as a child would to a parent without wondering if he would be welcomed."

—Sheila Walsh, *The Heartache No One Sees*

"The Lord is near to all who call on him, to all who call on him in truth."

—Psalm 145:18

Be confident in knowing that what you share here tonight and in future meetings will allow you to work through your own grief in your own way. This group will form bonds that will not be easily broken.

The most encouraging thing, as we begin our grief journey together, is knowing that God will be with us as we travel. We are never alone. And in our most desperate times, he carries us. While grief may haunt us, there is a time for it. Christ grieved. He knows the pain. Rest assured in the fact that God does have a blessed plan for your life...one that will allow you to flourish...one that will give you insurmountable blessings. We need to be open to receiving them.

The most encouraging thing, as we begin our grief journey together, is knowing that God will be with us as we travel. We are never alone.

Closing Prayer

Dear God,

Although we gathered here tonight as a group of grieving parents, we leave here tonight as a group that understands we are not alone. While you are always with us, Father, we sometimes feel as if we are the only person on earth who hurts this much and longs to hold children who are no longer here. Sometimes, it's comforting just to know that others can say "yes, I do understand." All of us here have known this pain. And as tragic as it is, we do thank you for bringing us together. We pray a special blessing on all of us here and pray that our hearts begin to mend and heal as we go through this journey together.

In Jesus' name,

Amen.

Week 1 Memory Verses

"'For I know the plans I have for you,' declares the Lord, 'plans to prosper you and not to harm you, plans to give you hope and a future.'"

—Jeremiah 29:11

"'You will seek me and find me when you seek me with all your heart.'"

—Jeremiah 29:13

Homework

❶ Write down what your plan for your life is. By this I mean, what your goals are/were and your time plan. What was your plan before your loss? What is it now?

_____

_____

_____

_____

_____

❷ Write down what you think God's plan for your life might be.

_____

_____

_____

_____

_____

❸ Compare the two. Does your timeline match his? Are your goals for yourself the same as his? Do you see any differences or similarities? Be prepared to share next week if you feel led to do so.

_____

_____

_____

_____

_____

❹ Read the Introduction and do Week 2 in preparation for next week's group.

Breaking the Silence

Giving Permission to Grieve

> *"Carry each other's burdens, and in this way you will fulfill the law of Christ...for each one should carry his own load."*
> —*Galatians 6:2, 5*

Opening Prayer

Dear God,

Thank you for giving us all the courage to come here tonight. We honestly seek your presence, guidance, love and comfort. We also ask that you guide our meeting tonight as we share our stories, our fears, our hopes and our grief with one another. Allow us to bear witness to each other's life in a way that allows us to carry each other's burdens. Thank you for carrying our burdens. Thank you for who you are and what you will do through this group.

In Jesus' name,

Amen.

Breaking the Silence

> *"Carry each other's burdens, and in this way you will fulfill the law of Christ...for each one should carry his own load."*
> —*Galatians 6:2, 5*

Silence. Silence so loud that my ears ached from it. There was no laughter, no cries, and no voices in the hall. Just hours before, the room where I lay was full of nurses, beeping machines, and shouts of instruction. Now, there was nothing.

After lying in the maternity ward in a labor and delivery room for two days, I was used to the hustle and bustle of welcoming new life into the world. I heard mothers screaming in pain, crying in joy, and laughing with delight at the first site

Silence. Silence so loud that my ears ached from it. There was no laughter, no cries, and no voices in the hall.

of their newborn. Suddenly, I was on a surgical recovery floor, at the end of a long, dark hall, in a still room where no noise was made or heard...just silence.

As I lay in my hospital bed, staring at the traffic out my window, I couldn't believe that the world was actually continuing. It had only been five hours since I had delivered my twins, stillborn at 22 weeks, into the world. I didn't understand why the world wasn't coming to a screeching halt. With desperation, I rationalized that since they did not know of my pain, they could not bear it with me. And so they would continue with their lives while mine was put on an agonizing hold. It would all continue in silence.

For those who did know of the pain and loss I had suffered, they offered me little comfort. Even those whom I knew loved me, and whom I loved as well, could not help me with this pain. Very little was even said.

It seemed that "mum's the word" was the theme that encompassed everyone who came to visit me. Some, especially family members, were also grieving the loss of my babies. After all, a twin pregnancy is an exciting event, and the thought of having identical twin girls running around was all anyone could talk about in the family. Now, nothing was said. Silence again.

While in the gazed trance of window staring, I heard the nurse talking to my parents and husband in the hallway.

"She needs closure. She already said good-bye to these babies when they were born dead. You need to help her let them go."

"How can we do that?" my mother asked.

"There's no need to discuss the babies anymore. Don't let her mind linger on this tragedy. Go home and pack up all the baby clothes. Don't make her go through the pain of having to put their things away. Let her get on with her life and put this behind her," the nurse replied.

Immediately, I remembered the two little mint green outfits I had bought the week before. They were tiny, trimmed in white satin around the neckline. There was even a little bear stitched on the pocket of each one. I began to cry at the thought of someone putting them in a box. Sadness turned into anger, and then, to silence.

When my mother, father and husband entered the room, I continued to stare out the window. Without looking away, making eye contact with any of them, or giving any inflection to my tone, I simply said "Despite any advice you've been

It seemed that "mum's the word" was the theme that encompassed everyone who came to visit me.

given, do not touch anything in the nursery. Do not open the door. If I go home and find one thing out of place when I get there..." Then I turned and looked at them all, my face conveying the meaning of my words, and I continued, "I will never forgive any of you for it." Not knowing any words to say, they simply nodded and sat down. Again, there was silence.

The rest of the nurse's advice was taken, my twins were never mentioned. If I dared to bring up the subject of them, the conversation immediately turned to something else. Even my father, who is naturally a man who lingers on crisis-at-hand issues, changed the topic when I began to comment on how they looked so much like my mother.

"For identical twins, they didn't look a thing alike to me. I think they both looked like Mom though."

"Yeah, you're right. I wonder what they are planning to do with all that fill-dirt piled up out there," he said.

Needless to say, I got the picture. And the room, once again, went silent.

By afternoon, I was exhausted from the silence. I was exhausted from everyone trying so hard to forget the one thing that I wanted to remember so much. So I decided that I would remember them by myself, in isolation, and I asked that no more visitors be allowed in the room.

That evening as darkness covered the landscape that I had stared at out the window all day, there was a knock on the door. My husband came to say that his family had been waiting for hours and would like to know if they could see me.

"No," I said quietly. "Ask them to leave."

"Christa's here," he said, "She's really wanting to see you...could she come in?"

The thought of Christa seemed to warm me. Christa was his sister. I had always loved her as a friend and as the "sister I never had." Feeling the need for some kind of sister-like encouragement and love, I told my husband I would like to see her. But everyone came in with Christa's invitation.

They all walked in the room in single file. First were my husband's parents, then his younger sister, and then Christa and her husband. They all huddled around my bed except for Christa. She leaned up against the wall as if she were patiently waiting for her turn to speak. I heard lots of "It's okay, they're with God now," and "the doctor said you can have more children." They expected that to bring me great comfort, but it didn't. After all the "comforting comments" were

> By afternoon, I was exhausted from the silence. I was exhausted from everyone trying so hard to forget the one thing that I wanted to remember so much.

spoken, silence once again filled the room. Everyone left, except Christa.

Slowly, she walked from her position against the wall and sat down on the chair beside my bed. She placed her purse that once hung from her shoulder in the center of her lap. She opened it and pulled out her wallet. Underneath her driver's license was a small, folded white piece of paper. Carefully, she unfolded it, making sure that it was not harmed in any way. She gently ran her fingers over it and with a warm smile, placed it in my hand. As I looked down at the tiny unfolded paper, I saw the Xerox copy of two tiny footprints.

"Here are my babies," she said. "Now, tell me about yours."

Suddenly, I remembered that this woman, this dear friend, had lost twins too. They had been stillborn at 23 weeks and she knew exactly what to do. She knew that the silence was drowning me in the grief and that it was time for her to send me a life raft.

All I could do was smile and cry. These were not tears of grief but tears of joy and relief. Tears of knowing that she knew how I felt and how badly I needed to talk about my children. We sat and talked for what seemed like days about how their little faces were beautiful and how the muscles on their legs looked so strong. We talked about how we knew that they would have been doctors, lawyers, writers, Nobel Peace Prize winners or even stay-at-home moms. It didn't really matter what dreams we held for them; all that mattered was that we had dreams for them. We knew they were special. We knew it wasn't wrong to talk about them, the dreams we had for them, or even the way we so desperately missed them.

After we laughed and cried, we prayed. We asked for God's grace over both of us. We asked Jesus to hold our babies' hands, because, for now, we couldn't. Somehow, that image alone produced great comfort. It wasn't simply hearing "they're with God now;" it was actually asking him to hold them. Again, they were real, not just a "sad thing that happened." They were my babies.

Encouragement, love, friendship and comfort like this doesn't come with detailed instructions. It comes with the faith that even though you might be going against popular advice and thought, you are doing what you know is best for your friend. Doing what God has led and called you to do. It

> Tears of knowing that she knew how I felt and how badly I needed to talk about my children.

is simply modeling his comfort. It is sharing one another's burdens through breaking the silence.

Christa knew me. She knew how I longed for the lives of these babies, and she knew that their death would not stop that longing. She knew that while I carried them for only a few months, I knew them as any mother knows her children. She knew that although they were not alive on earth, they would always be alive in me. She knew that not remembering them, not talking about them, would not do justice to them or to me.

And finally, the silence was broken.

Passage Comments

The story reflects my personal story with the loss of my children. So often, it is said that those who grieve "unknown children" grieve in silence. It was only when a dear friend of mine, who had also suffered the same grief, gave me permission to grieve the loss of my children that a burden had been lifted.

This brings us back to our scripture passage:

> "Carry each other's burdens, and in this way you will fulfill the law of Christ...for each one should carry his own load." (Galatians 6:2, 5)

Paul isn't "talking out of two sides of his mouth." Paul states bearing each other's burdens in this way to make a point. Those of us who are carrying "boulders" need help more so than those carrying a "knapsack" of burdens. Every person will carry his/her own knapsack of burdens into the room, and in their totality, the boulder of grief that each one shares will be carried by all. This group is centered on carrying each other's burden with love and encouragement in a horrifically difficult time...a time each one here is sharing. That is the purpose of this group. This group will love, encourage and most importantly LISTEN to each other in a way that no other group can, simply because everyone here is walking a similar path. Our stories will not match identically, but they do bear resemblance.

> Paul states bearing each other's burdens in this way to make a point. Those of us who are carrying "boulders" need help more so than those carrying a "knapsack" of burdens.

Discussion

 Talk about your own hospital experience. Was it similar to the author's? Explain.

_____

_____

_____

_____

_____

❷ What has been your family's/friends' reaction to the death of your child?

_____

_____

_____

_____

_____

❸ What do you wish their response would have been?

_____

_____

_____

_____

_____

❹ Had you ever known anyone else who had lost a child from miscarriage, still birth or early neonatal death? If so, what was your reaction to their loss?

_____

_____

_____

_____

_____

❺ Knowing now what you didn't know then, how has your perspective changed?

_____

_____

_____

_____

_____

❻ If you could tell the person beside you one thing about your child, what would it be?

_____

_____

_____

_____

The most reassurance you can find will come from knowing that Christ loves you and his heart breaks with your grief as well. His promise is encouraging, strong and hopeful, for his "yoke is easy and [his] burden is light" (Matthew 11:30). And, as always in your toughest walks of life, that is when he carries you.

Reflection

Take some time on your own, outside of the group time, to journal about your thoughts on this chapter.

_____

_____

_____

_____

_____

_____

_____

_____

_____

_____

_____

_____

_____

_____

_____

Encouragement

"Her story and the sorrow embedded in her eyes shook me. But one comment in particular unnerved me. 'Thank you,' she said, 'for letting me know it is not wrong to suffer.'"

—Dan Allender, *The Healing Path*

Closing Prayer

Dear Lord,

Thank you that you do not expect us to be silent, but you give us freedom to break the silence and talk about the babies we love…the babies you love. Comfort each of us now in our grief. In Jesus' name, Amen.

Week 2 Memory Verse

"Carry each other's burdens, and in this way you will fulfill the law of Christ…for each one should carry his own load"

—Galatians 6:2, 5

Homework

❶ Be a "Christa" to yourself. Write down your memories of your child(ren) to share with the group next week so that others here may become a "Christa" to you.

_____

_____

_____

_____

❷ Do Week 3 in preparation for next week's group.

Rollercoasters

Up and Down with Grief's Emotions

"Then Jesus went with his disciples to a place called Geth-semane, and he said to them, 'Sit here while I go over there and pray.' He took Peter and the two sons of Zebedee along with him, and he began to be sorrowful and troubled. Then he said to them, 'My soul is overwhelmed with sorrow to the point of death. Stay here and keep watch with me.'

"Going a little farther, he fell with his face to the ground and prayed, 'My Father, if it is possible, may this cup be taken from me. Yet not as I will, but as you will.'

"Then he returned to his disciples and found them sleeping. 'Could you men not keep watch with me for one hour?' he asked Peter. 'Watch and pray so that you will not fall into temptation. The spirit is willing, but the body is weak.'

"He went away a second time and prayed, 'My Father, if it is not possible for this cup to be taken away unless I drink it, may your will be done.'

"When he came back, he again found them sleeping, because their eyes were heavy. So he left them and went away once more and prayed the third time, saying the same thing."

—*Matthew 26:36-44*

Opening Prayer

Dear God,

Thank you again for bringing us all here safely. Please be with us and guide us through this meeting. Your presence is something we truly long for here. Keep our minds and hearts open to what you want us to hear and share. We pray for your love to hold and encompass us. Let your parental arms hold us as only a loving Father can. We know that you've experienced grief. We need your healing. We pray for that now for each one of us here tonight.

In Jesus' name,

Amen.

Rollercoasters

"Then he said to them, 'My soul is overwhelmed with sorrow to the point of death. Stay here and keep watch with me.'"

—Matthew 26:38

Rollercoasters. Life can be described as a rollercoaster ride. You know that feeling, the anticipation of getting to the top of the first big hill on the track. The big hill that gives the ride the momentum to carry on. The clink, clink, clink of the chains catching below the cars on the tracks lifting you up into the air only to have you plummet back again to the earth. For months, my rollercoaster was going down that first huge hill. That drop is supposed to be brief. That drop has a purpose. For me that drop was never ending. My life had become a constant fall, and I just kept waiting to hit the bottom.

I didn't really know what the bottom looked like. It couldn't look much worse than the fall. Sometimes it felt numbing. Sometimes it hurt so bad that I couldn't breathe. Sometimes I wondered what I should have done to keep from falling. What I could have done to make the ride go the way it was supposed to go. Sometimes I wondered why God put me on this ride in the first place. After all, wasn't he supposed to prevent the pain of the fall? Sometimes I was too angry to even care about falling or about the ride itself.

For me, the most frustrating part was that everyone else was telling me how to act while I was falling. People would try to explain to me that falling had a definite end. For many, it was an end that I should have already reached. Others had set a finite date in their mind and if I surpassed that date, then I was no longer a suffering mother, I was someone who "should have gotten over it by now."

I couldn't begin to fathom how the world carried on so smoothly in judgment while I was suffering so much. How could I be expected to function in society while I was falling? Frustration overwhelmed my very being because no one understood that while I didn't want to keep falling, I had no way of stopping it, and to simply "quit" or "get over it" was not an option.

> For me, the most frustrating part was that everyone else was telling me how to act while I was falling.

My next assumption was that I must be a failure. I couldn't stop the fall. It was my fault in the first place. But, then again, shouldn't the professionals who built and sustained the ride be held to blame since they should have predicted this? Where did God fit into this? Couldn't he have prevented the fall or even the ride itself in the first place? Or was the fall simply a punishment for something horrible I had done? The blame must be placed on someone. It was either me, the professionals or God. Obviously, someone had failed. And failure was not acceptable.

Anger took over. *Why was this happening? Why did it happen to me?* I wanted the ride to end. I wanted to go on with my life—WITH my baby. It wasn't fair. It wasn't just. It wasn't righteous. Other people have babies everyday who don't even want them. I wanted mine. But I couldn't have her. I wanted to demand justice! Why did other women get to see their children's names in the paper and I had to read mine on a tombstone?

Anger took over. *Why was this happening? Why did it happen to me?* I wanted the ride to end.

I even had thoughts of ending the ride altogether. I didn't want to be on the ride anymore. The never-ending pain of the fall was too severe. The fall would be worth it if I had a baby in my arms after I got off the ride, but I knew there was no baby there to hold. Getting out of bed each day became a chore and sleep was my only salvation. I could dream of my child. In my dreams she was alive again. Sadly, the world kept moving, even as I fell in my sleep.

Passage Comments

This rollercoaster analogy describes the beginning stages of my own journey of grief. The stages of grief were made popular by Elizabeth Kubler-Ross in her book *On Death and Dying*.

The stages of grief are:
1. **Denial**
2. **Anger**
3. **Bargaining**
4. **Depression**
5. **Acceptance**

Again, two things must be considered. First, it must be explained that the array of emotions one experiences while traveling through grief is not limited to these specific stages. However, these stages accurately represent the most common emotions in grief. The second notable reflection is that not everyone goes through these stages in order or at the same pace.

For example, the mother who's suffering from a recent loss might be lingering in stage two, while her husband is in stage four. It might take one person a month to go through the stages of grief while others could take a lifetime. Some may never complete all the stages.

Also, it must be understood that the stages of grief might be experienced in a different order than presented. A father who has recently suffered a loss might go from Denial to Bargaining and back to Denial again before experiencing Anger. There might also be a "pinball effect" where a grieving parent bounces back and forth between stages.

It is essential to remember that everyone's grief is unique. And a parent's grief is always valid. There is no time limit. There is no right or wrong way to grieve.

Also, it must be understood that the stages of grief might be experienced in a different order than presented.

Discussion

❶ Describe your rollercoaster.

_____

_____

_____

_____

_____

❷ The author wrote: "Sometimes I wondered why God put me on this ride in the first place. After all, wasn't he supposed to prevent the pain of the fall?" Do you believe that God is supposed to "prevent the pain"? Or do you believe he will equip you to persevere through the pain? Discuss your feelings and beliefs about this.

_____

_____

_____

_____

❸ Have you felt pressure regarding your pain to just "get over it"?

_____

_____

_____

_____

_____

❹ Have you, like the author, had thoughts of "ending the ride altogether"? Talk about those thoughts and feelings.

_____

_____

_____

_____

❺ What gives you strength to continue on?

_____

_____

_____

_____

❻ Have you felt guilty over the way you are grieving? If so, why do you think that is?

_____

_____

_____

_____

7 What stage of grief are you in currently? What stages have you already experienced?

_____

_____

_____

_____

_____

8 What have you found helps you most in working through your grief?

_____

_____

_____

_____

_____

Grief can at times be all encompassing. Jesus, himself, experienced this type of grief. He also experienced the loneliness that came along with it. Jesus was not experiencing the loss of a child, but the loss of his own life. He was also experiencing his most intense grief among those who claimed to love him the most and whom he certainly loved.

> We, as parents of dead children, wholeheartedly understand what that statement means.

Jesus said "My soul is overwhelmed with sorrow to the point of death" (Matthew 26:38). We, as parents of dead children, wholeheartedly understand what that statement means. So when you cry to your Savior for comfort as your soul is dying from sorrow, he knows exactly what you're saying. Allow him to comfort you.

Reflection

Take some time on your own, outside of the group time, to journal about your thoughts on this chapter.

_____

_____

_____

_____

_____

_____

_____

_____

_____

_____

_____

_____

_____

_____

_____

_____

Encouragement

"...the wound, which causes us to suffer now, will be revealed to us later as the place where God intimated his new creation."

—Henri Nouwen, *The Wounded Healer*

Closing Prayer

Dear God,

Thank you for being with us here tonight. Thank you for your wisdom. We ask special healing on those of us who still have open wounds from words others have spoken to us. Allow us to progress through the stages of grief in the manner best suited for us. Let us not care what others say about our grief progression. Let your will be done. Please dwell within us all and bring us back safely again next week.

Amen.

Week 3 Memory Verse

"Then he said to them, 'My soul is overwhelmed with sorrow to the point of death. Stay here and keep watch with me.'"

—Matthew 26:38

Homework

❶ Journal about the stage of grief you are experiencing and what you're expecting next. When doing this, envision the rollercoaster metaphor, and apply it to what you're currently experiencing and what you think is over the next hill.

_____

_____

_____

_____

_____

❷ Do Week 4 in preparation for next week's group.

The Blame Game

Placing the Blame on Those Who Caused Your Loss

"On his arrival, Jesus found that Lazarus had already been in the tomb for four days. Bethany was less than two miles from Jerusalem and many Jews had come to Martha and Mary to comfort them in the loss of their brother. When Martha heard that Jesus was coming, she went out to meet him, but Mary stayed at home.

"'Lord,' Martha said to Jesus, 'if you had been here, my brother would not have died.'

"And after she had said this, she went back and called her sister Mary aside. 'The Teacher is here,' she said, 'and is asking for you.' When Mary heard this, she got up quickly and went to him. Now Jesus had not yet entered the village, but was still at the place where Martha had met him. When the Jews who had been with Mary in the house, comforting her, noticed how quickly she got up and went out, they followed her, supposing she was going to the tomb to mourn there.

"When Mary reached the place where Jesus was and saw him, she fell at his feet and said, 'Lord, if you had been here, my brother would not have died.'

"When Jesus saw her weeping, and the Jews who had come along with her also weeping, he was deeply moved in spirit and troubled.

"Jesus wept.

"Then the Jews said 'See how he loved him!'"

—John 11:17-21, 28-33, 35-36

Opening Prayer

Dear God,

Thank you again for bringing us all here safely. Please be with us and guide us through this meeting. Your presence is something we truly long for here. Keep our minds and hearts open to what you want us to hear and share. As we talk about those we blame for the death of our children, let us show compassion. Let us know and understand that placing blame will not bring our children back to us and will only lead us to destruction. This might mean destruction of ourselves, our relationships with those we blame and even in our relationship with you. Lord, help us to move across the hurdle of blame. Heal us.

In Jesus' name,

Amen.

The Blame Game

"When Mary reached the place where Jesus was and saw him, she fell at his feet and said 'Lord, if you had been here, my brother would not have died.'

"Jesus wept."

—*John 11:32, 35*

Forgiving is often a struggle. Forgiveness for many means a simple "I'm sorry." For others it means seeing a result...a total turn around in behavior that inflicted distrust, disagreement or pain. Forgiveness is usually sought only after blame has been assigned.

We are all called to forgive, regardless of blame. Blaming is easy, forgiveness is not. As a Christian, sometimes forgiveness is a battle. As a mother of dead children, forgiveness is a war.

When my children died, I had so many people to blame. My own name topped the list. The race was a tight one, but God came in a close second. My husband, family and doctor then rounded out the top five. I took my shots at each one—one at a time.

I was the easiest of all the victims. Self-blame haunted me. Sleepless nights echoed with the words "Maybe if I hadn't..." At times, I couldn't decide which was worse—losing my children or knowing it had been my own fault. I relived every decision I had made from the choice of pregnancy test to oversleeping the morning my water broke. Like a professional

> Self-blame haunted me. Sleepless nights echoed with the words "Maybe if I hadn't..."

boxer, I took jab after jab until I lay in bloody defeat in the middle of the ring.

God was my next target. After all, he was the one who gave me these children, only to take them away again. How could a merciful God do such a thing? How could he sit back and quietly watch my children die? God never fought back. He just took the beating. My verbal thrashing was like a whip on his back. And like a slave servant, he withstood all the punishment.

After that, I began to reflect on the months prior to my babies' death. I remembered how tired I was, how sick I was. Still I had to do the housework. I still had to go to work every day. I still had to carry heavy loads of laundry up and down the stairs. Blame soon turned to anger toward my husband. After all, if he would have helped out more, this wouldn't have happened. He was as much to blame in the death of my children as I was...even more so. It also seemed as if he wasn't even grieving—he had taken everyone's advice and "gotten over it." *It!* Our babies were not "its!" I wondered how he could even sleep at night knowing that he killed our babies.

My family made jokes throughout my pregnancy. "Oh, you better get used to feeling bad all the time. Just wait "'til those twins get here. You'll never have any sleep! You'll be feeling terrible for the next two years!" Joke after joke was made about my horrible all-day morning sickness, my exhaustion and my size. Maybe now that my children are dead, the joke would end. If only they had been there for me, taken me seriously, helped me more. Isn't that what family is supposed to do? Obviously, if they would have been there for me, this would not have happened. My children would still be alive.

The doctor—well, my doctor was a very easy target. "You're gaining too much weight," I was told. "But I can't eat...I'm constantly throwing up!" I tried to plead. "Well, obviously, something's staying in or you wouldn't be so heavy," he joked. It wasn't until my water broke three weeks later and I watched my stomach deflate like a balloon that it was suddenly evident that all that was "staying in" was pounds and pounds of excess fluid. Had he only listened, had my medical coverage been better, maybe I would have gotten better medical care. And my babies would still be alive. I was convinced he was the devil incarnate. It was probably his plan all along to see my babies buried. What a horrible man.

> Blame soon turned to anger toward my husband. After all, if he would have helped out more, this wouldn't have happened.

With my blame list in tow, I went through years of accusations and branding, calling on each member's name on the list over and over again. Bitterness filled the spot where my children's lives should have been. My life had become as frigid as ice. Malignancy has a way of doing that. It wasn't until one warm April morning that things began to thaw....

Passage Comments

Blame is a logical part of grief. However, those we blame aren't always logical choices. Logic put aside, it doesn't make it any less real. Perception at this point is the griever's reality. It is key to really assess our blame.

While it has been said that blame is a logical part of the grieving process, it tends to be a tool of evil. Blame will sever relationships. It happens in marriages. It happens in our relationship with God. Blame will never bring your child back. Blame will never comfort or save you from your grief. That will come through forgiveness.

As I ended the story, you were left hanging. I discussed blaming and bitterness. I illustrated the coldness that both blame and bitterness can bring, and left you with the image of a thaw. What do you suppose will happen next?

> Blame will sever relationships. It happens in marriages. It happens in our relationship with God.

Discussion

❶ Name whom you blame for the death of your child.

_____

_____

_____

_____

_____

❷ Why do you place the blame there?

_____

_____

_____

_____

❸ How does this person respond to your blame?

❹ What do you wish this person's response would be?

❺ How has your relationship with this person been impacted by your blame?

❻ Have you ever considered that those on your "blame list" might not be aware that you hold them responsible? Do you think they understand why you blame them? Explain your answer.

❼ What is your response to forgiving this person?

_____

_____

_____

_____

_____

❽ Read Galatians 5:1, 13-15. Discuss what you think you could experience if you were to release yourself and others from your blame.

_____

_____

_____

_____

Jesus knew death and mourning. He also knew what it was like to be blamed for the death of someone whom he dearly loved.

As a parent, God has big shoulders. He tells us that his yoke is easy and his burden is light (Matthew 11:30). He will take our burdens and grief and bear them until we can take them back from him and carry them ourselves.

> As a teenage daughter, I blamed my mother for many things. I blamed her for everything that hurt me and that I couldn't control.

As a teenage daughter, I blamed my mother for many things. I blamed her for everything that hurt me and that I couldn't control. And she gladly took the blame, knowing that I was not strong enough to carry it myself. That's the character of a good parent. And God is the ultimate parent.

As a human, God knew the pain of grief. He wept. Can you see the Savior crying for his loss? Can you imagine Mary rushing to him, falling at his feet crying "if only!" Fall at Jesus' feet and allow him to mourn and weep with you.

Reflection

Take some time on your own, outside of the group time, to journal about your thoughts on this chapter.

_____

_____

_____

_____

_____

_____

_____

_____

_____

_____

_____

_____

_____

_____

_____

_____

_____

Encouragement

"'My name is *Bearing-the-Cost*, but some call me *Forgiveness*.'

"…She gazed at the little flower and said again, 'Why call you that?'

"Once more, a little whispering laugh passed through the leaves, and she thought she heard them say, 'I was separated from all my companions, exiled from home, carried here and imprisoned in this rock. It was not my choice, but the work of others who, when they had dropped me here, went away and left me to bear the results of what they had done.'

"'I have borne and have not fainted; I have not ceased to love, and Love helped me push through the crack in the rock until I could look right out onto my Love the sun himself. …He shines upon me and makes me to rejoice, and has atoned to me for all that was taken from me and done against me. There is no flower in all the world more blessed or more satisfied than I, for I look up to him as a weaned child and say, "Whom have I in heaven but thee, and there is none upon earth that I desire but thee.""

—Hannah Hurnard, *Hinds' Feet on High Places*

Closing Prayer

Dear God,

Thank you for being with us here tonight. We ask special healing on those of us who still have bitterness and blame lists of our own. Don't allow our anger or bitterness to consume the memories we have of our children. We ask that you give us forgiving hearts. Help us to fall at your feet, and give us eyes to see you weeping along with us. Please dwell within us all and bring us back safely again next week.

Amen.

Week 4 Memory Verses

"When Mary reached the place where Jesus was and saw him, she fell at his feet and said 'Lord, if you had been here, my brother would not have died.'"

—John 11:32

"Jesus wept."

—John 11:35

Homework

❶ Make your top 5 list of whom you blame for your baby's death and why. Then, determine your first step in forgiving each person. Be prepared to share it next session if you feel led to do so.

_____

_____

_____

_____

❷ Do Week 5 in preparation for next week's group.

Tasting Forgiveness

"But now you must rid yourselves of all such things as these: anger, rage, malice, slander, and filthy language from your lips."

"Therefore, as God's chosen people, holy and dearly loved, clothe yourselves with compassion, kindness, humility, gentleness and patience. Bear with each other and forgive whatever grievances you may have against one another. Forgive as the Lord forgave you. And over all these virtues put on love, which binds them all together in perfect unity."

—Colossians 3:8, 12-14

Opening Prayer

Dear God,

Thank you again for bringing us all here safely. Please be with us and guide us through this meeting. Your presence is something we truly long for here. Keep our minds and hearts open to what you want us to hear and share. Lord, please help us to offer forgiveness to those whom we feel are to blame for the death of our children...whether that be our spouse, our doctors, our employers, or even ourselves. Help us to be clothed in compassion, kindness, humility, gentleness and patience. Help us to show the same forgiveness to others that we have already received from you.

In Jesus' name,

Amen.

Note:

From this point, you may feel a wide range of emotions. You may feel hurt, sadness, anxiety, self-blame, anger, resentment and frustration. Forgiving those whom we've labeled as "faulty" in our child's death is a very hard thing to do. In our humanness, we want to hold onto that anger. Stay committed to prayer for each other (even silently) throughout the sessions...relying on the Lord to soften, and keep soft, each of your hearts, allowing them the capacity to forgive.

Tasting Forgiveness

"Bear with each other and forgive whatever grievances you may have against one another. Forgive as the Lord forgave you."

—*Colossians 3:13*

It was a beautiful April day. Warm, sunny, spring blooming outside. Yet inside it was still so very cold. Everything looked dark. No matter how brightly the sun shone, all I noticed were the shadows it would cast.

It was a Friday. There was a special church service that night and my husband had to read Scripture. I didn't want to go. I hated seeing everyone there. People still felt awkward around me...not knowing how to act or what to say. And I resented them for it.

The service was going smoothly, as it usually did. I stared blankly at the stained-glass windows, not caring to be there...or anywhere for that matter. A foul taste filled my mouth as I heard the hymns praising him for who he was. I felt like throwing up. I still wondered where God had been six months earlier when my children died—why he didn't care that I was in so much pain.

My theological perspective began to get even more tainted as I sat in the pew that night. I began to tell God that I was fed up with his attitude. I screamed through silent tears, If you could only understand! And why weren't you there for me?!?! I was so alone. No one knew my pain. Frankly, no one tried.

So I continued to sit there. Stone. A crying statue. No sounds. No noise. Only silent tears. My trance was broken by my hearing what sounded like a calf being slaughtered. I looked up to see my husband sobbing loudly behind the pulpit. Emotion flooded his words. At first, shocked, all I could do was stare...then, finally, I listened.

"They spit on him, and took the staff and struck him on the head again and again. After they mocked him...they led him away to crucify him."

> I still wondered where God had been six months earlier when my children died—why he didn't care that I was in so much pain.

It was Good Friday. They were reading the passion story from Matthew and Luke. The words began to soak into my skin like oil as he continued, "'Father, forgive them, for they know not what they do'" (Luke 23:34, KJV). The words were like a slap in the face. I sat, awestruck, motionless. John's sobbing became more intense as he read on screaming, "'My God, my God, why have you forsaken me?'" (Matthew 27:46). His words were so real, emotions so raw. We were both living that moment together. We had both felt forsaken.

Suddenly, I realized what I had been missing for so long. God spoke to me so very clearly that night. He, too, had lost a child. He lost his only child. His child was sinless, the ultimate sign of hope and promise. He watched his child die. It was his plan, no matter how painful. And in the midst of the pain, in the midst of bearing the sins of the world, he pled, "Father, forgive them."

There were so many, many people to rightfully blame. Peter and his disciples denied him. Judas handed him over. Pilate allowed the crucifixion, knowing Jesus was blameless. The people cried out "Crucify him!" and his Father watched as he blamelessly bore the sins of the world. And yet...Jesus...Jesus begs "forgive them." Suddenly, I realized I had been the one shouting "Crucify! Crucify! Crucify!"

My heart broke again that day. I felt I had let everyone down, especially the One who loved me the most. Bitterness had taken over the beautiful, albeit brief, experience I had with my children. Remembrances of feeling them move inside me quickly led to a feeling of hatred toward my husband for not taking each opportunity offered to place his stomach on my abdomen to feel it with me. I had not paid homage to their memory. I had used it as a springboard for hate and disgust.

I made a pledge that day. I pledged to God, myself, and my children, that I would not allow my babies' memory to be tainted. I promised to remember them in love...to thank God for allowing me to know them. To thank him for the lessons this would teach me, even though I could not see or understand them yet. I promised to live again. More importantly, I promised to seek to forgive, just as I was forgiven.

> God spoke to me so very clearly that night. He, too, had lost a child. He lost his only child.

Passage Comments

Spiritually, I turned away from God during my struggle of grieving my babies. This segment was a turn back in the right direction. I realized that blaming was putting me in a downward spiral that would only result in more death.

In the realm of spiritual warfare, we seem to have a clear-cut case of Satan on the attack. While it has been said that blame is a logical part of grief, one must ask "what does blaming accomplish?" Spiritually, all it accomplishes is more death. Satan sits back and feeds off your anger yelling "Crucify, Crucify, Crucify." It's now time to go on the offense against the enemy and offer forgiveness...just as you were forgiven.

Discussion

❶ What has your attitude toward God been since the death of your child?

_____

_____

_____

_____

_____

❷ In dealing with your grief, can you give examples where blaming someone has hurt you even more?

_____

_____

_____

_____

❸ When we have someone to blame, we may feel that our life isn't totally out of control. If you didn't have someone you could blame, how would you feel? Like your situation is out of control?

_____

_____

_____

_____

_____

We want answers, especially relating to tragedy. Blaming helps us to feel like there's an answer—an explanation for our painful situation. Trusting that God is still in control and that he is good can allow us the freedom to release blame.

❹ On the scale below, indicate to what extent you are able to release the blame and live by faith that God is good and knows what he is doing.

1	2	3	4	5

Completely Unable   *Completely Able*

Forgiveness and trust are things that are not possible with our human tendencies. They come when we take on the model and sufficiency of Christ.

❺ Describe what you think your life would be like if you were to forgive everyone that you now blame, give your confusion to God and trust that he knows what he is doing.

_____

_____

_____

_____

_____

Reflection

Take some time on your own, outside of the group time, to journal about your thoughts on this chapter.

_____

_____

_____

_____

_____

_____

_____
_____
_____
_____
_____
_____
_____
_____
_____

Encouragement

"To excuse what can really produce good excuses is not Christian charity; it is only fairness. To be a Christian means to forgive the inexcusable, because God has forgiven the inexcusable in you."

—C. S. Lewis

"Forgiveness does not change the past, but it does enlarge the future."

—Paul Boese

"Forgiveness brings freedom—freedom from being controlled by the past, freedom from the emotional ties to the offender, freedom from the continual inner conflicts of bitterness and hate, freedom to become whole and enjoy the fullness of life."

—Jeanette Vought

"A rattlesnake, if cornered, will sometimes become so angry it will bite itself. That is exactly what the harboring of hate and resentment against others is—a biting of oneself. We think that we are harming others in holding these spites and hates, but the deeper harm is to ourselves."

—Eli E. Stanley

Closing Prayer

Dear God,

Thank you for being with us here tonight. Thank you for your mercy and forgiveness. We ask special healing and guidance to those of us who are struggling with the issue of forgiveness. We also ask that you forgive us for any sins we've committed in our anger, bitterness and resentment. Lord, help us in showing forgiveness to those whom we feel have sinned against us, trusting that even our painful circumstances are not out of your faithful, good control. Bless us as we refill our thoughts with loving memories of our pregnancies and babies and their lives with us, albeit too brief. Please dwell within us all and bring us back safely again next week.

Amen.

Note:

This is likely to have been a very powerful session, and may also be very confusing. You are dealing with your grief and loss as well as your own guilt. This is quite a mix! You might feel resistance or frustration if you are not yet able to reach forgiveness in your grief. Remember, everyone's grief is unique. Everyone reaches the stages of grief at his or her own pace. I encourage you to trust the Lord's leading in your life and be open to the biblical truth of forgiving others as the Lord has forgiven you. May the Lord bless your courage and faith.

> You might feel resistance or frustration if you are not yet able to reach forgiveness in your grief. Remember, everyone's grief is unique.

Week 5 Memory Verse

"Bear with each other and forgive whatever grievances you may have against one another. Forgive as the Lord forgave you."

—Colossians 3:13

Homework

 From the list you made last week, try praying for each of these people. If possible, communicate with them discussing your progress within the group. If you feel you're at a point of forgiveness, write each of them a letter expressing your feelings, thoughts, and disappointments. After it's complete, using safety precautions, immediately burn it. This signifies a "wiping away" and represents the end of a hold this person had on you. Afterward, journal about your feelings about the letter, about burning the letter, about your feelings after having burned the letter, and then journal about what God has done in your heart regarding forgiveness of this person and trust in him.

_____

_____

_____

_____

_____

❷ Do Week 6 in preparation for next week's group.

Grief Discrimination

When Others Don't Validate Your Suffering

"Jesus said, 'Father, forgive them, for they do not know what they are doing.' And they divided up his clothes by casting lots."

—Luke 23:34

Opening Prayer

Dear God,

Thank you again for bringing us all here safely. Please be with us and guide us through this meeting. Your presence is something we truly long for here. Keep our minds and hearts open to what you want us to hear and share. Please comfort us, Lord, when we feel alone and invalidated. Please help us to show understanding when others are ignorant of our grief and lack compassion. May we be so loving as to show compassion to them.

In Jesus' name,

Amen.

Grief Discrimination

"Jesus said, 'Father, forgive them, for they do not know what they are doing.' And they divided up his clothes by casting lots."

—Luke 23:34

"Oh, I just feel so sorry for her. My heart breaks for her every time I think about it. It's just not fair that her baby is gone."

I heard this while sitting alone in a restaurant one afternoon. My booth was directly across the aisle way from the conversation. As I overheard this one sentence, I just had no recourse but to look up and follow this conversation.

Her friend, sitting across from her in their booth continued, "I know, I know. I'm so glad that our church family was able to get dinner ready for them in the fellowship hall for after the funeral. It's so important to support them now. That poor young girl is grieving herself to death."

Immediately, I wanted to jump up and say, "Who is she?" or "I'm grieving for my baby too...maybe we can support each other." But I sat and listened...staring into my full plate of untouched food.

The first lady responded, "Well, what can you expect? She was only a day old. They had no idea that anything like this would happen...I mean, it's not like she miscarried...she actually held her baby and saw her. She was told all along that their little girl was fine. Her doctor never caught it. Can you imagine how awful that must be for her?"

My heart sank. Tears welled up in my eyes as I began to feel like I was choking. I hadn't eaten a bite but something was welling up in my throat. It was as if I was suffocating. I immediately got up and ran to the restroom. I sat in the handicapped stall and cried. Finally, it had all become so very clear as to why the world was reacting to my loss. Finally, these ladies had verbalized what I had feared all along.... My grief wasn't as "significant" or "valid" as this other mother's.

Ironically, as I sat there, I began to wish I was the other mother. I wished I could have held my baby for an hour...or two. I can't imagine being able to look upon her face for a whole day! I even wished I could have gone through the hours of labor and birth she got to experience in anticipation of holding the baby at the end...not knowing that something horrible was about to happen...only knowing that my suffering with childbirth would end with a live cry. I even wished I would have the sympathy that came along with her tragedy...instead of the type that didn't come along with mine.

Was this other mommy also suffering? Certainly. Was her pain as intense or as horrible as mine? Absolutely. Was I in any way downplaying her pain? No way.

You see, I've been on both sides of that fence. I've held 22 week old babies, lifeless and still. I've also lost babies at 7 and 9 weeks. Both experiences are horrible. Both carry tremendous amounts of pain. Both are real. Both are significant. All are valid.

> I wished I could have held my baby for an hour...or two. I can't imagine being able to look upon her face for a whole day!

All these babies mattered to their parents. All these babies mattered to God. All were precious. All are irreplaceable...to all those who loved them.

Passage Comments

The sad fact of the matter lies in the fact that most of the time, you can't change other people's beliefs. Someone usually has to go through something first hand to experience it's reality. I can honestly say that my mind could not have fully comprehended the severity of this type of loss had I not experienced it myself. And if we're all completely honest with ourselves, our reactions would have been the same as the rest of the population. This is why we need each other for support.

Furthermore, we also need to move to understanding. Ignorance is not an excuse, but it is an explanation. As the old adage says, you don't know what it's like until "you walk a mile in another man's shoes." If we can take on an attitude of understanding in our grief, then we are truly modeling Christ's example.

> If we can take on an attitude of understanding in our grief, then we are truly modeling Christ's example.

During Christ's ultimate betrayal, he said "forgive them, for they know not what they do." They lacked understanding, sympathy, love. Christ's only communion was with his Father. Now, you not only have that blessed assurance, but you also have the fortunate experience to have the support of those who have "walked in your shoes."

Discussion

❶ What is your personal reaction to the author's story?

_____

_____

_____

_____

_____

❷ Have you "walked in her shoes"? Share your experience.

_____

_____

_____

_____

_____

❸ What do you think the author means when she says "Ignorance is not an excuse, but it is an explanation"?

_____

_____

_____

_____

❹ What are your own feelings about "rating grief"? Do some parents have more of a "right" to grieve than others?

_____

_____

_____

_____

❺ How have your answers to question #4 changed since your own loss? Since you began meeting with this group?

_____

_____

_____

_____

❻ Has meeting with the group changed your feelings or beliefs in any way? Was it a change that could have been experienced any other way? Explain.

_____

_____

_____

_____

_____

One of the most comforting and encouraging passages to me came from Romans 8:26:

"In the same way, the Spirit helps us in our weakness. We do not know what we ought to pray for, but the Spirit himself intercedes for us with groans that words cannot express."

Sometimes we hit a wall of grief. There is a total sense of loss, loneliness and hopelessness. It is in these times when the Holy Spirit, the ultimate Comforter, comes to us and helps us. When our minds are haunted with nothing but the memory and longing for our child, "the Spirit himself intercedes for us with _groans_ that words cannot express" (emphasis added).

> Sometimes we hit a wall of grief. There is a total sense of loss, loneliness and hopelessness.

❼ As you allow yourself to grieve, what comfort do you find from Romans 8:26? Do you hear him interceding for you? Can you hear his groans that symbolize your pain and need for healing? Be still and listen.

_____

_____

_____

_____

_____

Reflection

Take some time on your own, outside of the group time, to journal about your thoughts on this chapter.

_____

_____

_____

_____

_____

_____

_____

_____

_____

_____

_____

_____

_____

_____

Encouragement

"Wounded people who have been broken by suffering and sickness ask for only one thing: a heart that loves and commits itself to them, a heart full of hope for them."

—Jean Vanier, founder of l'Arche

Closing Prayer

Dear God,

Thank you for being with us here tonight. We pray a special prayer for ourselves as well as all those who are suffering from the loss of a child. We pray for those who do not understand our grief. Give us compassion and understanding for them. May you continue to help us heal. And may the wounds in our own lives serve to help others heal as well. Please dwell within us all and bring us back safely again next week.

Amen.

Week 6 Memory Verse

"In the same way, the Spirit helps us in our weakness. We do not know what we ought to pray for, but the Spirit himself intercedes for us with groans that words cannot express."

—Romans 8:26

Homework

❶ Read Romans Chapter 8. Reflect on Romans 8:26. Journal about what this section means to you.

_____

_____

_____

_____

_____

❷ Do Week 7 in preparation for next week's group.

Finally! Validation At Last!

The Joy When Others Validate Our Grief & Place As A Parent

"Therefore, remember that formerly you who are Gentiles by birth and called 'uncircumcised' by those who call themselves 'the circumcision' (that done in the body by the hands of men)—remember that at that time you were separate from Christ, excluded from citizenship in Israel and foreigners to the covenants of the promise, without hope and without God in the world. But now in Christ Jesus you who once were far away have been brought near through the blood of Christ.

"For he himself is our peace, who has made the two one and has destroyed the barrier, the dividing wall of hostility, by abolishing in his flesh the law with its commandments and regulations. His purpose was to create in himself one new man out of the two, thus making peace, and in this one body to reconcile both of them to God through the cross, by which he put to death their hostility. He came and preached peace to you who were far away and peace to those who were near. For through him we both have access to the Father by one Spirit."

—Ephesians 2:11-18

Opening Prayer

Dear God,

Thank you again for bringing us all here safely. Please be with us and guide us through this meeting. We long for your presence here. Keep our minds and hearts open to what you want us to hear and share. Lord, we pray for your wisdom for both ourselves and for others. We thank you for your hope and for your love.

In Jesus' name,

Amen.

Finally! Validation At Last!

"...remember that at that time you were separate from Christ, excluded from citizenship in Israel and foreigners to the covenants of the promise, without hope and without God in the world."

—*Ephesians 2:12*

After I had traveled down the road to and from disbelief, anger, resentment, guilt and forgiveness, I continued to revisit them again and again. I began to wonder why God wouldn't just take them away. I read about Paul's "thorn" in his flesh. I began to wonder if my thorn was my grief. I tried to pluck it out so many times. All I ended up doing was digging into my flesh, making it raw. The thorn remained and the flesh around it was tattered and mangled.

Life, of course, continued. I fell into a regular routine. *Work, home, bed. Work, home, bed. Work, home, bed.* That was my life. Weekends were horrible. At least at work, I had something to do to keep me busy. At home, while I tried to do normal, everyday tasks, I felt drained and tired. I had decided to try to "live again" and while moments of laughter and happiness did come, they were fleeting and I usually ended up even more tired.

One weekend in particular, my mother called me and asked me for a favor. I told her I was still in my pajamas, but she explained to me that she had accidentally forgotten her glasses and needed them. So I told her I would bring them within the hour.

I remember that morning very clearly. My husband was attending a Promise Keepers breakfast at our church. I was alone and, of course, lonely. I remember looking at our bookshelf that morning and seeing the twins' baby books. They were still empty. I had a few personal reminders of them that I kept in a beautiful purple box with a satin tie. I kept it on my nightstand close to me. But the empty baby books haunted me too. They lived, if only inside of me, but their books showed nothing.

I walked by the bookshelf as I went to get dressed and ran my fingers along the books as a child does with a stick on a fence. I left the house and went to get my "mother's" glasses, and then to our town's local family-owned shoe store. It was a busy Saturday afternoon with several people buying spring sandals.

Life, of course, continued. I fell into a regular routine. *Work, home, bed. Work, home, bed. Work, home, bed.* That was my life. Weekends were horrible.

My mother was standing at the counter speaking with an elderly lady. As I walked up, I noticed that I recognized the lady as being a frequent customer I had seen on several occasions. My mother reintroduced me to her. "And this is my youngest child, Sylvia." I just smiled.

"With three children, you must have a lot of grandchildren by now," the lady said to my mother.

Immediately, my mother responded, "Yes, I have seven." Then said with a giggle and a wink to the lady, "And they're all perfect too. I'm not biased or anything either."

Suddenly, I ran the numbers through my head. My oldest brother only had one child. My other brother had four. That only totals five.

I began to choke up. The other two...the other two...were my babies. She had remembered them. They were in the seven. They were her grandchildren too. They counted!

I took my mother's hand, and with tears running down my face, I quietly said, "Thank you." Mom just smiled. Finally, validation. She understood...and did all along. However, it wasn't until that moment that I understood. It was in that moment, by her response to a simple question that she was able to show me that my grief was authenticated, and that she loved my children too.

> Mom just smiled. Finally, validation. She understood...and did all along.

I believe, in that moment, my mother plucked the thorn from my side. My husband had felt the pain of grief too. While he understood my grief, the social stigma of and toward pregnancy loss confined him from making any "declarations" of our children. Hearing that my children were one of my mother's grandchildren showed me that they had lived. That was priceless. I went home that day and filled out their baby books. Only the first few pages are complete. The pages about the first weeks, first tooth, first step and first day of school are marked with the words "In heaven...will report later." Again, hope with validation...what a beautiful thing.

Passage Comments

We all have our thorns. Sometimes grief becomes our weakness as we allow it to consume the very nature of who we are. There is a time for everything. There is a time for grief. Everyone's grief is unique and should be treated accordingly. Grief isn't a one-time thing. It's a process where we can go through stages repeatedly and stay in one stage for a while. This is normal and acceptable.

I needed to know that their lives mattered, that they mattered.

Seeking validation in our grief is also acceptable. However, oftentimes we don't ask for it or find it. Oftentimes, we don't even realize that's what is holding us in our grief. For me, not only did I grieve the loss of my children, but I also grieved the loss of their importance to others. I needed to know that their lives mattered, that they mattered. What a true mark of a mother!

Discussion

❶ What things validate grief (i.e. funerals, memorials, others' sympathy)?

_____

_____

_____

_____

_____

❷ Did you receive these things?

_____

_____

_____

_____

_____

❸ What could be done now that would break the silence of "disallowed grief"?

_____

_____

_____

_____

_____

❹ Has your grief become your "thorn"? If so, what do you think it will take to remove it?

_____

_____

_____

_____

_____

5 If your thorn is grief, have you tried unsuccessful methods of removal? What were they and what were the results?

_____

_____

_____

_____

_____

6 Is validation of your grief important to you? Why or why not? Explain your answer.

_____

_____

_____

_____

_____

7 Do you feel your grief has been validated? If so, please explain to the group how.

_____

_____

_____

_____

_____

Jesus, being perfect, grieved, as we've read earlier in this book. He faced great loss, and his grieving was valid, just as yours is valid. God promises us hope beyond our grief. Sometimes hope is all we think we have. But remember, *ALWAYS*...these three remain: faith, hope and love. But the greatest of these is love. Even if we're hopeless, God never is. And above all, he loves you. Just as you love your child.

Reflection

Take some time on your own, outside of the group time, to journal about your thoughts on this chapter.

_____

_____

_____

_____

_____

_____

_____

_____

_____

_____

_____

_____

_____

_____

Encouragement

"We often hear that brokenness is the pathway to a deeper relationship with God, but we rarely see it modeled. I sometimes think we want others to believe that we know God by demonstrating how unbroken we are."

"But we've all been wounded."

"...Something brilliant and intact gleams through the stain of our brokenness."

—Larry Crabb, *The Safest Place on Earth*

Closing Prayer

Dear God,

Thank you for hope. Thank you for your love. Thank you for being our Father. Please be with us all here tonight who are still seeking validation of our grief and for those of us who are still seeking to break the silence of that grief. We pray for grace. We pray for the understanding of those with whom we come into contact and especially for those whom we hold most dear. Allow us to share with them the words that we need to share and allow them to understand and love us as we need to be loved. Father, we know that you are the one who loves us the most, and again, we thank you for that. Please be with us this week and bring us back safely next week.

In Jesus' name,

Amen.

Week 7 Memory Verse

"...remember that at that time you were separate from Christ, excluded from citizenship in Israel and foreigners to the covenants of the promise, without hope and without God in the world. But now in Christ Jesus you who once were far away have been brought near through the blood of Christ."

—Ephesians 2:12-13

Homework

 If you haven't already, purchase a baby book and fill out what you can in it. Or, write in a notebook or on your home computer a memorial to your baby. Include things such as:

- When you found out you were expecting

- How you told your spouse / How your spouse told you

- What was your and your spouse's initial reaction
- Who you told
- What his/her reaction was
- The day of your baby's death
- Any other information you would like to include

❷ Do Week 8 in preparation for next week's group.

Words Like Swords

When People Say Hurtful Things

'reckless words pierce like a sword, but the tongue of the wise brings healing."

—Proverbs 12:18

Opening Prayer

Dear God,

Thank you again for bringing us all here safely. Please be with us and guide us through this meeting. Your presence is something we truly long for here. Keep our minds and hearts open to what you want us to hear and share. As we talk about words that hurt or have hurt us, let us be filled with your Spirit and forgiveness. Thank you for your grace, and may we also show that grace to others.

In Jesus' name,

Amen.

Words Like Swords

'Reckless words pierce like a sword, but the tongue of the wise brings healing."

—Proverbs 12:18

Two years after I lost my babies, my pastor approached me with a question.

"What do I say to these people?"

He went on to explain that he had been called that very morning. The voice on the other end of the line explained that she was in town on business for a couple of months and had gone into premature labor. Her baby had died during birth. She did not know our pastor, or anyone personally in town. It was only she and her husband. She picked our pastor's name blindly out of the phone book.

She was seeking a pastor to do her son's burial service. "Nothing fancy," she explained to him. "Just something for him. To remember him." Our pastor and his wife were expecting their first child. He was young and new to the ministry and had only done a couple of funerals. To him, this seemed to be an insurmountable task.

After his explanation, he asked again, "What do I say? How can I comfort them?"

His last question made me chuckle. My giggle made him nervous. I think I offended him, embarrassed him and scared him all at the same time. Of course, from my perspective, it made perfect sense. My viewpoint clearly illustrated the ridiculousness of his probe. To me he was asking "How can I be God to them?" Now, our pastor is a wonderful, righteous man, but...he's certainly no Jesus.

I went on to explain that there is very little that he could say or do. And, in all reality, his best bet was to say nothing. "Words are too often like swords," I explained. "They can be helpful at times, but can also cut very deep. They are also very dangerous."

He listen and agreed. In a very considerate tone he asked, "What should I say at the funeral?"

I simply smiled. Oh, how I wish the pastor from two years ago had sought such counsel. I almost envied this grieving mother for having found a pastor who put aside his fears, embarrassment and pride, and sought words of wisdom from experience. With these thoughts, I lowered my head and choked back the tears, allowing only one to escape. I simply said, "Say that she knew this child. That he was loved. And that he would always have a mother who loved him."

"All right. I understand," he replied. After a little bit of silence and thought, he continued, "What shouldn't I say?"

Immediately, I relived my babies' funeral. The words of the pastor echoed in my head. "No one knew these children, Father, but you knew them, even in the womb." What a horrible, horrible thing to say. I knew these children. I felt them move. I held their warm, lively bodies for five months. Then I held their cold, still bodies for a few precious hours. I knew them very well. And I could tell you right now, years later, without a moment's hesitation, any detail of their little bodies you would need to know. I could tell you every second of every ultrasound...when I could identify them readily before

> I simply said, "Say that she knew this child. That he was loved. And that he would always have a mother who loved him."

the nurses could. Their blurry images on a small screen that was produced by sound waves was like a window showing me their personalities, features, size, shape. I already knew my children. And I knew them very well. What an insulting thing to say to a grieving mother.

I also began to revisit the days following their death. "You can always have other children," I was told. "It's for the best. God has a plan," was another common response. One of the most hurtful was "Be thankful. At least you didn't go full term only to have them die." Another painful comment was "You have your whole life ahead of you." Some really did, in all sincerity, try to offer hope. "They're in heaven now," was a favorite among my church family. All I wanted to do was yell, "I don't want them in heaven...I want them here with me!"

"Sylvia?" he said, snapping me back to the present.

"Don't say anything to try to make her understand why this happened to her. Fight that urge. Don't try to offer any hope for her future. Simply let her grieve. And, tell her you know she loved her son, he would always be a part of her, and you're available to listen to her anytime she wants to talk about her experience or her precious baby."

When Pastor Dave got up to leave that day, I began to realize even more that as a parent who has suffered such a loss, we have a vital obligation. Words can cut like swords. Words echo in our minds at night when it's dark and sleep eludes us. It is our duty to help others minister to those who have lost their children to miscarriage or stillbirth. It is our duty to educate them. Imagine how wonderful it would have been not to have heard those ill-mannered, flesh piercing words from those who thought they were offering hope. Wouldn't it be a wonderful gift to give to other grieving parents?

> "Don't say anything to try to make her understand why this happened to her. Fight that urge. Don't try to offer any hope for her future. Simply let her grieve.

Passage Comments

There are two things that are critical about hurting words. The first is that most are unintentional. The second is that they usually come from those whom you love the most. This literally makes them a "double-edged sword."

Most of the most hurtful words spoken to me were by those in my church. These were the same ladies who had seen me grow from a four-year-old child into a woman and peer. I knew these ladies would never intentionally hurt me. But their words were not said prayerfully or with thoughtful consideration. They left gaping wounds in my flesh that were raw and sore. In reflection of the words of Proverbs, there was no "wisdom" in their tongue.

It is the wise man, and in this case, the wise pastor who seeks advice in speaking to mothers and fathers who have suffered the loss of a child. This pastor had the foresight to understand that no words he spoke could heal the parents and nothing he could do would take away their pain. What he also knew was that his words could hurt far more than he could comprehend. He allowed his confidence, human wisdom and knowledge of God's word to be put aside, and he sought advice from someone who had walked in the grieving parents' shoes. He allowed God's wisdom to work through him by listening to a woman who had felt the pain that came with hearing the wrong words. And he was a much wiser man for it.

Discussion

❶ What are some of the hurtful words that you've heard since your baby's death?

_____

_____

_____

_____

❷ What were some of the words you wish you had heard?

_____

_____

_____

_____

❸ Speculate at what stage of grief the author was experiencing. Support your speculation with details.

_____

_____

_____

_____

_____

4 How many weeks, months or years do you believe had passed since the author had experienced the death of her babies?

_____

_____

_____

_____

_____

5 What leads you to this conclusion?

_____

_____

_____

_____

_____

6 Do you agree with the author's declaration that we "have an obligation" to help other grieving parents? Why or why not?

_____

_____

_____

_____

_____

7 If you agreed with her declaration, how do you think we can fulfill our obligation?

_____

_____
_____
_____
_____

8 Are you at the point where you can fulfill this obligation? Why or why not?

_____
_____
_____
_____

9 Thinking back to the author's story, what advice would you have given the pastor?

_____
_____
_____
_____

As with all things, God offers
healing.

Proverbs offers us much in the way of wisdom. So often, we reflect on this week's memory verse as being about intentional words that are meant to hurt a person. Here, we can see that sometimes those who love us the most and want us to heal the most are the ones who deliver the wound. As with all things, God offers healing. If you think of healing in the physical realm, you know that God can heal all wounds. Allow God to heal the gaping wounds that hurtful words have left in your flesh. Rest assured that time doesn't heal all wounds. Again, that's God's job.

Reflection

Take some time on your own, outside of the group time, to journal about your thoughts on this chapter.

_____

_____
_____
_____
_____
_____
_____
_____
_____
_____
_____
_____
_____
_____

Encouragement

"In timeless words that have calmed the over-whelming fears of His children down through the centuries—fears that have threatened to...silence their voices, paralyze their feet, erase their minds, break their hearts, and destroy their faith, Jesus said with quiet authority, "Do not let your hearts be troubled" (John 14:1)."

—Anne Graham Lotz, *My Heart's Cry*

Closing Prayer

Dear God,

Thank you for being with us here tonight. Thank you for your wisdom. We ask special healing on those of us who still have open wounds from words others have spoken to us. We also ask that you forgive us of our trespasses as we forgive those who have trespassed against us. Please dwell within us all and bring us back safely again next week.

Amen.

Week 8 Memory Verse

'reckless words pierce like a sword, but the tongue of the wise brings healing."

—Proverbs 12:18

Homework

❶ Write down all the phrases that were so hurtful to you. After each one, write down what you wish had been spoken. If needed, follow the last statement with a statement of forgiveness.

For example:
Words said — "You can always have more children."
Wished Words — "I'm sorry your child died. I know you loved him/her."
"I forgive you, Karen, for saying these words. I know you would never intentionally hurt me."

❷ Do Week 9 in preparation for next week's group.

Healing Doesn't Mean Forgetting

Times When We Remember Our Babies

"When the hour came, Jesus and his apostles reclined at the table. And he said to them, 'I have eagerly desired to eat this Passover with you before I suffer. For I tell you, I will not eat it again until it finds fulfillment in the kingdom of God.'

"After taking the cup, he gave thanks and said, 'Take this and divide it among you. For I tell you I will not drink again of the fruit of the vine until the kingdom of God comes.'

"And he took bread, gave thanks and broke it, and gave it to them, saying, 'This is my body given for you; do this in remembrance of me.'

"In the same way, after the supper he took the cup, saying, 'This cup is the new covenant in my blood, which is poured out for you.'"

—*Luke 22:14-20*

Opening Prayer

Dear God,

Thank you once again for bringing us here tonight safely. Father, we've come a long way from our first week together and we thank you for walking with us through the journey. Please open our hearts and minds throughout these next stages in our lives so we can learn from you and each other. Father, we look forward to the day when we can remember our babies with smiles, instead of tears. We pray that you continue to bless us with your presence here again tonight as you have at our past meetings.

In Jesus' name,

Amen.

Healing Doesn't Mean Forgetting

"And he took bread, gave thanks and broke it, and gave it to them, saying, 'This is my body given for you; do this in remembrance of me.'"

—*Luke 22:19*

This past October was my twins' eleventh birthday. I only have a picture in my mind's eye of what they would look like now—or should I say "who" they would look like now. As parents of our children, it's our privilege to imagine what they would look like on whatever birthday rolls around. Parents are like that. Anniversaries are similar, when they roll around, they trigger our minds to stroll down the road of "what if."

For me, anniversaries come and go throughout the year that remind me of my girls. I think of them around their due date in February. Valentines hearts remind me of the cute little matching red jumpsuits I had looked at in preemie sizes made especially for the Valentine's Day baby.

I always think of them on June 17th, the day I got that first positive pregnancy test. Then again on the 18th when I got the second, third and forth positive pregnancy tests (yes, I was skeptical and shocked).

Falling leaves, pumpkins, and the smell of cinnamon spice remind me of the day that I had to say a final good-bye to them. Smelling fall leaves and hearing them crunch under my feet remind me of rushing into a hospital foyer asking where to go for the maternity floor. Ironically, I still get the "baby itch" (as my husband calls it) around the same time every year when I ponder whether I want to try again to have another child. It wasn't until two years ago, 9 years after the twins' death, that I made the connection...same time every year...still looking to fill empty October arms.

Mother's Day, a day that should be celebrated and honored, is always hard. I love my living children. I also love and remember my dead children. I always remember my first Mother's Day without a living child. I always remember my first Mother's Day after my son was born. It's always bittersweet.

Of course, I can't help but think of them every time I see twin girls who look like they would be about the same age as mine. It always brings tears to my eyes. And I can never fight the temptation to remind their mother of how lucky she is to have her two beautiful little girls. You'll notice the same re-

Falling leaves, pumpkins, and the smell of cinnamon spice remind me of the day that I had to say a final good-bye to them.

sponse when you see children the same as your baby, especially if they share the same birthday as your due date. Being flooded with emotions of "if only" will lead you to relive your longing all over again. Sometimes it will be sad, and rest assured, other times will be happy....simply because you had the privilege of knowing your baby because you conceived him and carried him in your womb.

It used to make me feel guilty to have so many anniversary occasions that reminded me of them, their lives and their deaths. I used to think that if I really healed from my loss and overcame the grief, I wouldn't have so many triggers. But it became obvious to me that healing doesn't mean forgetting.

Jesus reminds us that it's okay to remember what is important to us—what is significant to us. He shows us that through remembering, we can be stronger and we can move on stronger. He told his disciples to remember him and to commune with each other in honor of him. Heal from the pain of his leaving, but delight in the hope of his return, and remember who he was and why he came.

> Jesus reminds us that it's okay to remember what is important to us—what is significant to us.

Healing means growing and living. It means remembering in a way that honors who we loved so dearly. It doesn't mean blocking out. It doesn't mean ignoring. It doesn't mean replacing. It doesn't mean preoccupation. And it certainly doesn't mean forgetting.

Passage Comments

Healing after a loss is oftentimes consuming. It's usually a long, uphill battle to overcome an all-consuming grief. Each day, each step leads us toward healing. Once we get to the top of the hill, slipping back down it again racks us with fear and guilt. When one loses a child, grieving does not stop. The intensity of the grieving often lessens as healing takes place; however, healing is often linked with forgetting. Forgetting our children, though, would not give honor to their memory.

Discussion

❶ What anniversaries make you think of your child?

_____

_____

_____

❷ What emotions do you experience with those memories?

_____

_____

_____

_____

_____

❸ Are you at peace with those emotions?

_____

_____

_____

_____

_____

❹ What does healing mean to you? What does it look like?

_____

_____

_____

_____

_____

❺ Has your perception of healing changed since your loss? Explain.

_____

_____

_____

_____

_____

6 Do you think others can understand the concept of "healing doesn't mean forgetting"? If not, why? And, if not, how can we help them to understand?

_____

_____

_____

_____

_____

7 All of us have experienced death in our lives, although not everyone has experienced the loss of a child. How do the two compare?

_____

_____

_____

_____

_____

8 Can "general loss" be used to help others understand that "healing doesn't mean forgetting"? Explain.

_____

_____

_____

_____

_____

Remembering your child is okay. Even years after your child's death it's still okay. Never let anyone tell you that it's time to forget or that it's time to "move on."

"Moving on" for those of us who know and who've suffered the loss of a child means walking through every day, one step at a time, until the time comes when we're reunited in heaven and can hold our child's hand. For now, we'll have to rest in the assurance that our child is in the glory of heaven and Jesus is holding his hand.

Reflection

Take some time on your own, outside of the group time, to journal about your thoughts on this chapter.

_____

_____

_____

_____

_____

_____

_____

_____

_____

_____

_____

_____

Encouragement

"The children hung a tiny stocking on the mantelpiece along with theirs. They now have a new treasure in heaven, known and loved and cared for by the Lord. Someday they will know her too. 'Where your treasure is, there will your heart be.'"

—Elisabeth Elliot

Closing Prayer

Dear God,

Thank you for being with us here tonight. Thank you for your love and healing. We ask special healing for those of us who are still traveling through heavy grief. We also ask for the healing of us who still experience guilt from ourselves or ridicule from others when we remember our baby. Give us and others understanding that healing is not forgetting. We also ask that you forgive us of our trespasses as we forgive those who have trespassed against us. Please dwell within us all and bring us back safely again next week.

Amen.

Week 9 Memory Verse

"And he took bread, gave thanks and broke it, and gave it to them, saying, 'This is my body given for you; do this in remembrance of me.'"

—Luke 22:19

Homework

❶ Holidays and anniversaries that remind us of our babies will, at times, revive grief. Map out a plan for those that you feel will be the hardest.

For example:

"I'm dreading Mother's Day because of how our church celebrates it during services, and I'm afraid that my congregation will feel awkward around me...or even worse, will forget that I'm a mother too. So I will go to another church in a surrounding area. I will also do something positive to remember my baby like planting a flowering shrub in my front yard. I will also treat myself to a late lunch at a new restaurant that I normally wouldn't try."

_____

_____

_____

_____

_____

❷ Do Week 10 in preparation for next week's group.

Lessons Learned

11 Years of Life Since I Met My Babies

> *"'For I know the plans I have for you,' declares the Lord, 'plans to prosper you and not to harm you, plans to give you hope and a future. Then you will call upon me and come and pray to me, and I will listen to you. You will seek me and find me when you seek me with all your heart. I will be found by you,' declares the Lord, 'and will bring you back from captivity. I will gather you from all the nations and places where I have banished you,' declares the Lord, 'and will bring you back to the place from which I carried you into exile.'"*
>
> *—Jeremiah 29:11-14*

Opening Prayer

Dear God,

Thank you again for bringing us all here safely. Thank you for these past weeks of study, sharing, exploring, and understanding. Thank you for all the times when we shared and for those times when we could not. We thank you for your love and for bringing us full circle in this group. We started in Jeremiah and we will end there as well. Thank you for bringing us back from the bonds of grief. While we still may be grieving the loss of our children, we will not be controlled by it because we know you will carry us back from the exile. Please allow us to have open minds and open hearts as we share again tonight.

In Jesus' name,

Amen.

Lessons Learned

"'Then you will call upon me and come and pray to me, and
I will listen to you.'"

—*Jeremiah 29:12*

Eleven years ago, I saw a glimpse of heaven. It came in the form of two small bodies. The epitome of perfection. Eleven years ago, I felt the pain of hell. It came in those same little bodies. A total separation from hope. Eleven years ago, I felt the pain of original sin. Eleven years ago, I felt the promise of eternal life. Eleven years ago, I couldn't fathom there was a lesson to be learned. Eleven years ago, the very idea seemed cruel. Today, I'm learning lessons everyday. Today, I thank God daily for teaching them to me.

Some of the lessons I learned are short. Some are long. Some lessons I learned almost immediately. Others I'm still learning today. And I'm confident I will learn more tomorrow. They all make sense. They are also lessons I could not have learned any other way.

"What are those lessons?" is the question I've been asked so many times by parents hurting from the same loss. These parents seek to find some kind of hope. Hope that there is a light at the end of their tunnel. These are strong Christian men and women who do truly love God. They understand his word. They seek it in their lives daily. Sadly, the enemy seeks them even more eagerly, planning to destroy their relationship with hope when they need him the most.

To answer their questions, I give practical life applications. The very first lesson I learned was that all life was valuable. All life counted. All life mattered. Life is a precious thing and is something to be held onto knowing that it can be gone as quickly as it came. I love my children...living and dead. I could never have loved them the way I do had I not suffered the life and death of my babies. Children are a gift—not a right, nor an inconvenience. What an incredible gift God gave me in this lesson!

I learned that no matter how strong I thought I was, I was only as strong as my weakest link. But I also learned that in my weakest link, he is made strong. I learned to lean on God not only in those intense first days and months, but also on those cold October mornings for the many years to come.

Mostly, I understood for the very first time how much God loved me, because I understood what it was like to have a child. I never knew that kind of love. I had wonderful parents

> The very first lesson I learned was that all life was valuable. All life counted. All life mattered.

myself. I already knew what it was like to HAVE unconditional love, but I never understood what it was like to GIVE it. For the first time, I understood what sacrificial love felt like because I would have gladly, wholeheartedly, traded my life for theirs so that they might live. Again, what a beautiful gift in that lesson.

Passage Comments

In my story, I talked about an unconditional love that I had never experienced. While I had received it from my own parents, I never understood the other side of it until I carried my own child. It took the connection that I developed with my own child to understand the love that God had for me as he sent his son, Jesus, to die for me. Of all the lessons I learned, this was probably the most valuable to me.

I also talked about the value of life and how precious a child is. Seeing parenting the life of a child as a privilege and not a right is something that even the best Christian might tend to ignore. It takes a loss like yours to fully understand these lessons. While it still might be hard to understand and hard to face, you will be blessed by these lessons.

Discussion

❶ What are some lessons you've already learned/are learning?

_____

_____

_____

_____

_____

❷ Would you have learned these any other way?

_____

_____

_____

_____

❸ Why or why not?

_____

_____

_____

_____

_____

❹ Have you learned any lessons from your group members? If so, explain.

_____

_____

_____

_____

_____

❺ Tell other group members about what you are thankful for from going through this CarePoint group.

_____

_____

_____

_____

_____

❻ Name the one thing you want others in this group to remember about you and your child.

_____

_____

_____

_____

_____

It seems that I went through all the stages of grief, experiencing all the emotions that went along with it. I found my Savior in the middle of that grief. Now, while I have forgiven and accepted the death of my children, I have never forgotten them. The experience made me stronger, and I've relayed the promises that I found to you....

God promised me early on that the plans he had for me would never harm me...but, they would make me prosper. Here I am today, an educated woman. I've been educated scholastically, emotionally, spiritually. This is an education written by God for me. He had no other students in mind.

The promise I leave with you is this...Everything in your life will work for good if you love God. If you seek him, you will find him, and if you pray to him, he will listen. This is not my promise. It is his. I promise that while the pain is fresh and new, lessons will be hard to see. With time, his lessons will be revealed to you. In his time, your gaping wounds will heal. But don't believe that time heals all wounds. That's God's job. And that's a job that he's perfected.

What a wonderful promise. What wonderful hope.

> The promise I leave with you is this...Everything in your life will work for good if you love God.

Reflection

Take some time on your own, outside of the group time, to journal about your thoughts on this chapter.

_____

_____

_____

_____

_____

_____

_____

_____

_____

_____

_____

_____

_____

_____

Encouragement

"But if you lean toward heaven, it leans back."

"It comes down to whether we are inviting and embracing the input and influence of God in the midst of our journey. Darkness is never completely dark when the light of God breaks through."

—Kathy Troccoli, *Live Like You Mean It*

Closing Prayer

Dear God,

Thank you for the lessons you allow us to learn through our tragedy. We ask special healing on those of us who still struggle with learning and seeing the lessons you give us. Sometimes it's hard for us to understand that you will work good through all things. Forgive us for that and grant us wisdom. Remind us daily that we can call upon you and you will listen. Thank you for allowing us these weeks to get to know each other and share with each other. Thank you for sharing our burdens. Thank you for those here who shared our burdens too. I pray that you take all of us in your arms and continue to walk with us through our grief until we can one day reflect back on our memories with our children as precious and not painful. Allow each one of us to carry your light of love, forgiveness and mercy into the world as we help others break the silence of grief.

Amen.

Week 10 Memory Verse

"'Then you will call upon me and come and pray to me, and I will listen to you.'"

—Jeremiah 29:12

Homework

❶ Read Romans 8. Paul gives us lots of promises and instruction. Write down what's most significant to you at this point in your grief and why.

_____

_____

_____

_____

_____

❷ Reflect on the lessons you've already learned.

_____

_____

_____

_____

❸ Live each day in remembrance of your baby and honor that memory while honoring your commitment to God to live for him.

Where to Go for Help

The fact that you're here, right now, is a wonderful step. Support groups are a wonderful way to work through your grief and to begin the healing process. More importantly, you realize that you are not alone! Everyone here is suffering the pain and grief of losing a child too.

Searching the World Wide Web

As previously mentioned, the internet age has opened us to a wide array of communities. The list below, though not by any means exhaustive, gives websites that might offer good information or support to those suffering from the death of a child through miscarriage, stillbirth and early neonatal death.

http://www.bellaonline.com/Site/miscarriage

http://www.aplacetoremember.com/

http://www.hannah.org/

http://www.griefshare.org/

http://www.silentgrief.com/

http://www.mend.org/home_index.asp

http://www.pain-heartache-hope.com/

http://www.angels4ever.com/

http://3littleangels.org

http://www.peacebears.org/home.html

Books

The following is a list of recommended books to assist parents who are grieving their dead child after miscarriage, stillbirth or early neonatal death:

Empty Arms: Coping After Miscarriage, Stillbirth and Infant Death. Sherokee Isle.

Empty Cradle, Broken Heart: Surviving the Death of Your Baby. Deborah L. Davis.

Empty Cradle, A Full Heart: Reflections for Mothers and Fathers After Miscarriage, Stillbirth or Infant Death. Christine O'Keeffe Lafser.

A Silent Sorrow—Guidance and Support for You and Your Family. Ingrid Kohn, Perry-Lynn Moffitt, Isabelle A. Wilkins.

Life Touches Life: A Mother's Story of Stillbirth and Healing. Lorrain Ash, Christiane Northrup, MD (Foreword).

Silent Grief: Miscarriage—Finding Your Way Through the Darkness. Clara H. Hinton.

We Were Gonna Have a Baby But Had an Angel Instead. Pat Schwiebert and Taylor Bills. An excellent book for the children in your life affected by the grief of the loss of your baby (your own children, nieces, nephews, cousins, etc.). Also touching for a grieving parent.

Organizations

You can find support, information and understanding from the following organizations:

- **MEND (Mommies Enduring Neonatal Death).** www.mend.org

- **Hygeia Foundation, Inc. Institute for Perinatal Loss and Bereavement.** www.hygeia.org

- **The National Stillbirth Society.** www.stillnomore.org

October 15—Sharing Information and Spreading Hope

National Pregnancy and Infant Loss Remembrance Day

In 1988, Ronald Reagan signed a proclamation, claiming October as "Pregnancy and Infant Loss Awareness Month." This began the first step in recognizing the grief, anguish and need for educating the public on those suffering from the loss of a child.

In 2001, 35 States had signed a resolution claiming October 15th as National Pregnancy and Infant Loss Remembrance Day. As of 2003, 39 states in total have signed. Those states still absent from the proclamation include: Alabama, Arizona, Colorado, Georgia, Illinois, Maryland, Montana, Vermont, Washington, West Virginia and Wyoming.

Please visit http://www.october15th.com/.

Light a candle at 7 p.m. (in your own time zone) on this day in remembrance of your own child as well as the other

parents' children. Pink and blue ribbons are worn throughout
the day as memorials and tributes to our children.

References

Friedman, Rochelle & Bonnie Gradstein. *Surviving Pregnancy Loss*. Boston: Little Brown & Co., 1982.

Goldback, K. R., D. S. Dunn, L. J. Toedter, and J. N. Lasker. "The effects of gestational age and gender on grief after pregnancy loss." *American Journal of Orthopsychiatry*. 61 (3): 461-67, 1991.

Kirkley-Best, E. and K. R. Kellner. "The forgotten grief: A review of the psychology of stillbirth." *American Journal of Orthopsychiatry*. 52: 420-429, 1982.

Kubler-Ross, Elizabeth. *On Death and Dying*. New York: Macmillan, 1969.

Lasker, J. N. and L. J. Toedter. "Acute verses chronic grief: The case of pregnancy loss." *American Journal of Orthopsychiatry*. 61 (4): 510-22, 1991.

Lasker, J. N. and L. J. Toedtler. "Predicting outcomes after pregnancy loss: Results from studies using the Perinatal Grief Scale." *Illness, Crisis & Loss*. 8(4): 350-72, 2000.

Potvin, L., J. N. Lasker and L. J. Toedter. "Measuring grief: A short version of the Perinatal Grief Scale." *Journal of Psychopathology and Behavioral Assessment*. 11: 29-45, 1989.

Prigerson, H. G. (et. al.: MK Shear, SC Jacobs , CF Reynolds, PK Maciejewski, JR Davidson, R Rosenheck, PA Pilkonis, CB Wortman, JB Williams, TA Widiger, E Frank, DJ Kupfer, C Zisook). "Consensus criteria for traumatic grief. A preliminary empirical test." *Psychiatry*. 174: 67-73, 1999.

Stinson, K., J. N. Lasker, Lonmann, and L. J. Toedter. "Parents' grief following pregnancy loss: A comparison of mothers and fathers." *Family Relations*. 41: 218-223, 1992.

Toedter, L. J., J. N. Lasker, and J. M. Alhadeff. "The Perinatal Grief Scale: Development and initial validation." *American Journal of Orthopsychiatry.* 58: 435-449, 1988.

Toedter, L. J., J. N. Lasker, E. M. Jassen. "Death Studies." 2001. 25: 205-228, 2001.

Zisook, S., R.A. Devaul, and M. A. Click, Jr. "Measuring symptoms of grief and bereavement." *American Journal of Psychiatry.* 139: 1590-1593, 1982.

Printed in the United States
153844LV00001B/51/P